LEADING CARDIOLOGISTS PRAISE
DR. ROBERTS AND *THE TRUTH ABOUT STATINS*

"This book is being published not a moment too soon. A global campaign is being launched for entire populations to consume statin drugs as antidotes to cardiovascular disease. No voice is as well informed as that of Dr. Barbara Roberts for setting the record straight and for educating the public on this life-affecting issue."

—Bernard Lown, M.D.
Cardiologist, Brigham and Women's Hospital, Boston
1985 Nobel Peace Prize recipient
Professor Emeritus, Harvard School of Public Health

"Statins have been shown to reduce the risk of cardiovascular disease but they are not without a downside. Dr. Roberts' book presents the other side of the statin story, the side-effect story, a story that many patients do not hear from their doctors. She reminds us that we have very few longterm studies of these drugs and that we must be aware of their side effects before we follow the advice of some advocates and put statins in the water."

—Paul D. Thompson, M.D.
Medical Director of Cardiology
and the Athletes' Heart Program
Hartford Hospital, CT

Also by Barbara H. Roberts, M.D.

———

How to Keep from Breaking Your Heart:
What Every Woman Needs to Know
about Cardiovascular Disease

THE TRUTH ABOUT STATINS

Risks and Alternatives to
Cholesterol-Lowering Drugs

Barbara H. Roberts, M.D.

POCKET BOOKS
New York   London   Toronto   Sydney   New Delhi

Pocket Books
A Division of Simon & Schuster, Inc.
1230 Avenue of the Americas
New York, NY 10020

The ideas, procedures, and suggestions in this book are intended to supplement, not replace, the medical advice of trained professionals. All matters regarding your health require medical supervision. Consult your physician before adopting the medical suggestions in this book, as well as about any condition that may require diagnosis or medical attention. The author and publishers disclaim any liability arising directly or indirectly from the use of this book.

First Pocket Books paperback edition May 2012

POCKET BOOKS and colophon are registered trademarks of Simon & Schuster, Inc.

For information about special discounts for bulk purchases, please contact Simon & Schuster Special Sales at 1-866-506-1949 or business@simonandschuster.com.

The Simon & Schuster Speakers Bureau can bring authors to your live event. For more information or to book an event contact the Simon & Schuster Speakers Bureau at 1-866-248-3049 or visit our website at www.simonspeakers.com.

Designed by Julie Schroeder

Manufactured in the United States of America

10 9 8 7 6 5 4 3

ISBN 978-1-4516-5639-8
ISBN 978-1-4516-5640-4 (ebook)

In memory of my mother,
Dorothy Hudson
1922–2010

CONTENTS

Part 3: A Closer Look at the Science

Part 4: The Safe, Delicious Statin Alternative

INTRODUCTION

Statin medicines to lower cholesterol were approved in the United States in 1987. Over the last few decades, I have been prescribing statins for my patients when it was indicated, and, initially, these medicines seemed safe and reasonably well tolerated. But the more I have learned about statins, both from the experiences of my own patients and in the medical literature, the more concerned I have become. As more and more people have taken statins, there have been more and more reports of serious and sometimes fatal side effects. Now that statin use has accelerated, I feel compelled to share the results of my research into this powerful class of medicines. By educating readers about the facts behind the supposed miracle cure, I hope to encourage you to speak freely with your medical practitioners and to make informed decisions about preserving your heart's health.

Every day, in my practice as director of the Women's Cardiac Center at the Miriam Hospital in Providence, Rhode Island, I see patients who cannot tolerate statins. Some of them complain about muscle aches and weakness, or tendonitis, while others struggle with frightening memory loss and difficulty concentrating.

These side effects may not be as rare as we've been led to believe.

In fact, my husband developed severe muscle pain from every statin on the market. He was started on statins after a trip we took to Italy in 1995, when he more or less overdosed on prosciutto di Parma. He came home to a total cholesterol count of over 300. His primary care doctor prescribed various statins over the years, but his muscle aches interfered with his ability to run and lift weights, which he loves to do. Finally, he went on the seafood-vegetarian Mediterranean diet that I describe in this book. His cholesterol levels, from this diet and a nonstatin medicine that blocks the absorption of cholesterol, are now satisfactory.

Some people can take statins and not develop side effects. But how necessary are statins in the first place? Do they really help prevent strokes and heart attacks? Nowadays, doctors are advised to knock down their patients' cholesterol to very low levels with high doses of statins. But cholesterol, far from being the villain it's said to be, is a vital part of every cell in our bodies. This waxy fat, produced primarily by the liver, is absolutely crucial for the normal functioning of muscles, nerve cells, and the brain—and it's also the building block that our bodies use to manufacture many hormones, including the reproductive hormones estrogen and testosterone. How will our muscles, brain cells, and nerves react if they are chronically starved of a chemical that is so necessary for their proper functioning?

These and other important questions about statins need unbiased, scientifically valid answers. Why do women seem to derive less benefit from statins than men do? Why do women report more side effects from statins? What questions should you ask your doctor if he/she wants you to take a statin? How solid is the science that is used to justify treating people with statins? What is now at stake for the pharmaceutical industry (Big Pharma), the US Food and Drug Administration (FDA), the medical profession, and, most important, the people who take statins?

In researching these issues, I pored over the studies that were used to justify treating people with statins. I spoke to my own patients who'd experienced side effects from the drugs, and to other people who'd heard of my interest in statin side effects and contacted me. I educated myself on the interactions among Big Pharma, the FDA, and the medical profession.

The FDA is responsible for reviewing and approving any new prescription drugs that pharmaceutical companies want to sell to the American public. When this approval process is complete, the government agency spells out the specific reasons (*indications*) why doctors may prescribe the drug. The drug label must describe the approved reasons to use the medicine, along with the conditions under which the medicine should not be used (*contraindications*). For example, taking statins is contraindicated in pregnancy because these drugs can cause defects in a developing fetus .

The FDA not only certifies all new prescription drugs but also must approve *any new use of existing drugs*. However, once the FDA approves a drug, physicians can prescribe it for anything they choose. Unapproved indications are called *off-label* uses of a drug. Doctors can prescribe, but pharmaceutical companies cannot advertise, off-label uses of a drug.

Statins are approved to treat high levels of *low-density lipoprotein (LDL) cholesterol* (so-called bad cholesterol). In most cases, they are prescribed for people with high levels of cholesterol or with built-up fatty deposits called *plaque* in their *arteries*: those who either have or are at risk for *atherosclerotic cardiovascular disease* (ASCVD). Several scientific studies found that statins lowered the risk of cardiac events in people with established *atherosclerosis*. (*Events* is the neutral term we doctors use for really bad outcomes like heart attacks and death.) However, the benefit was modest and was less in women than in men. Furthermore, despite statin therapy, people with ASCVD still had a high residual risk—that is, they had an increased risk of heart attack and stroke even when their LDL cholesterol was brought to very low levels. There were also studies that showed benefits of statin therapy in people *without cardiovascular disease* but with elevated levels of LDL cholesterol. This benefit was found only in men, however, not women.

In February 2010, based on a study called the JUPITER trial, the FDA expanded the indication for statin use. It now included healthy men ages fifty and older and healthy women ages sixty and older—even those with normal levels of LDL cholesterol—if they have evidence of inflammation in the body (indicated by elevated levels of a substance called *high-sensitivity C-reactive protein,* or *hsCRP,* in the bloodstream), plus one other risk factor for developing heart disease, such as smoking or high blood pressure. *JUPITER* is an acronym for Justification for the Use of Statin in Prevention: An Intervention Trial Evaluating Rosuvastatin. This new indication for rosuvastatin (Crestor), the statin used in the trial, could add six and a half million *healthy* people—who exhibit no evidence of ASCVD and have normal cholesterol levels—to the number taking statins.

The trial recruited close to eighteen thousand people who were free of diagnosed heart disease. Half were treated with rosuvastatin and half received a *placebo,* or inactive "dummy" pill. The people enrolled in the study were then followed for the occurrence of cardiovascular events such as nonfatal heart attacks, stroke, or death due to cardiac disease, or the need for coronary artery bypass surgery or other procedures to improve blood flow to the heart.

The trial was scheduled to last five years but was stopped prematurely "for benefit" after an average follow-up of just under two years. This means that the investigators felt that the benefit of the statin in lowering the risk of cardiovascular events was sufficient to end the trial before it was scheduled to end. So based on the results of this study, the FDA approved wider use of rosuvastatin.

The JUPITER trial was paid for by AstraZeneca, the pharmaceutical company that makes Crestor. The principle investigator, Dr. Paul Ridker, developed the blood test that measures hsCRP, and he receives royalties from its use. Both AstraZeneca and Dr. Ridker stand to make a fortune as this new indication for statin use is implemented.

But are the results of this study all they are cracked up to be? Might the findings have been different if the JUPITER trial lasted five years, as originally specified? Was the FDA correct in approving this new indication for rosuvastatin? Were there differences in the results for women compared to men? The answers to these questions may shock you and make you question your physician if he or she wants to put you on a statin.

In exposing the shoddy science that underlies many of the "guidelines" that doctors are told they must follow in treating their patients, and in exposing the rampant conflicts of interest among the FDA, Big Pharma, medical scientists, medical centers, and professional medical organizations, I risk being declared a pariah in the medical community.

But this story must be told. If you or someone you love takes a statin, please read this book. It might just save your life.

Part 1

ARE STATINS
FOR ME?

Chapter 1

My Doctor Wants Me to Take a Statin—What Questions Do I Need to Ask?

Mrs. R.G. is a forty-five-year-old woman who is in good health. She has a yearly checkup with her primary care doctor, who has told her that she needs to lose weight. She works full time as an accountant and has two teenage children. She also cares for her parents, who are in their late seventies and chronically ill: her mother with severe arthritis and her father with blindness from macular degeneration. With little time for exercise, she has gained thirty pounds since graduating from college. She also "de-stresses" by eating cookies and candy. Her most recent cholesterol numbers reveal that her total cholesterol is 255, her triglycerides (another blood fat) are 200 (normal is up to 150), her HDL, or "good," cholesterol is 50, and her LDL, or "bad," cholesterol is 165.

Her doctor tells her to go on a low-fat diet and prescribes the statin drug simvastatin (brand name, Zocor) to get her LDL cholesterol down. Within two weeks of starting this medicine, she has severe muscle pain and difficulty concentrating. She goes online and looks up statin side effects. Convinced that she is suffering adverse effects from the simvastatin, she calls her doctor, who orders a blood test to look for muscle damage. The test comes back normal, so her doctor tells her that the statin is not causing her symptoms. Mrs. R.G. stops the statin anyway, and within a few weeks, her muscle pain and difficulty concentrating are gone.

A Brief Primer on Cholesterol

What is cholesterol, and why do we need to be concerned about it if the level is considered high? If your doctor tells you your cholesterol is 250, for example, what does that mean?

In addition to being manufactured in the body, cholesterol is also found in foods derived from animal sources. Cholesterol serves many important functions in our bodies. It's an integral part of the cell membrane that surrounds every cell in our bodies, keeping all the structures inside the cell from leaking out. It is a building block of other molecules that our bodies need to function, such as vitamin D, and many hormones. Cholesterol is used to make bile acids, which assist in digestion.

Cholesterol circulates in the blood bound to special proteins called *lipoproteins,* which are classified according to their density. (*Lipos* is a Greek word meaning "fat.") So LDL cholesterol is low-density lipoprotein cholesterol ("bad cholesterol"), and HDL cholesterol is high-density lipoprotein ("good cholesterol"). VLDL cholesterol, made up mostly of triglycerides, is very-low-density lipoprotein that, when elevated, increases the risk of ASCVD. Taken together, these lipoproteins are referred to as blood fats or blood lipids. Although cholesterol is absolutely essential for life, high levels of certain lipoproteins (and low levels of HDL cholesterol) can be harmful because they increase the risk of developing plaque in the arteries, the blood vessels through which oxygenated blood reaches all the body's cells. Atherosclerosis, the name for this process, underlies most heart attacks and strokes.

Our lipoprotein levels are determined both by our genes and by our lifestyles. For example, people who consume diets that are high in starchy carbohydrates will often have high triglyceride levels. Those who eat large amounts of animal fat (found in meat and dairy products such as milk, butter, and yogurt) will often have high levels of LDL cholesterol. There are some people with a rare familial form of high cholesterol who have very high levels of LDL cholesterol even if they are strict vegetarians.

How Cholesterol Is Measured

Cholesterol and triglycerides are usually measured on a fasting sample of blood. You will be told to fast for twelve hours. (You may drink water but should not eat or drink anything that has calories.) A blood sample will be taken and then spun in a centrifuge to separate the red blood cells from the clear part of the blood (plasma). The plasma will then be analyzed by a machine that measures the total cholesterol, the triglyceride level, and the HDL cholesterol. The level of

LDL cholesterol is then calculated using a formula. (It can be measured directly, but this is generally not done unless the triglyceride level is very elevated, because in that instance, the calculated LDL cholesterol level is inaccurate.)

The cholesterol values are reported as milligrams per deciliter, abbreviated mg/dl. A gram is a unit of weight, and a milligram is one-thousandth of a gram. A potato chip weighs about 1 gram (1,000 milligrams), so you can see that we're talking small quantities here. A deciliter is one-tenth of a liter, or about 3 ounces of liquid. So a total cholesterol level of 250 mg/dl means that there is an amount of cholesterol weighing about the same as one-quarter of a potato chip in 3 ounces of plasma.

Evidence-Based Medicine

The patient described at the beginning of this chapter is a composite drawn from many people I have seen in my office over the years. Throughout this book you will read the stories of actual patients who have been harmed by statins, but I used Mrs. R.G. as an example of the patients I often see who are put on statins even though they do not meet the current guidelines for using these medicines. Nowadays, doctors are urged to practice what is called "evidence-based medicine." In other words, we are urged to use only those medicines or procedures that have been proven by scientifically valid clinical research studies to have more benefits than risks.

In chapter 7, I will discuss the somewhat checkered history of clinical research, but to simplify a complex subject for the purposes of this chapter, when and how to treat cholesterol, based on the best available scientific evidence, is spelled out in the Adult Treatment Panel III guidelines from the National Cholesterol Education Program (NCEP), established by the National Heart, Lung, and Blood Institute. Unfortunately, the guidelines are published in lengthy articles that the average doctor is too busy to read in detail. Many doctors read that the "optimal" LDL cholesterol is under 100, and they come away feeling that anyone whose LDL cholesterol is over that number should be on medicine. The upshot is that many people are taking statin medicines unnecessarily, and a significant proportion of them are being harmed.

Among the well-known side effects of statins are muscle pain and inflammation, and damage to many other organs, including the liver, tendons, nerves, and the brain. And since cholesterol is essential for the normal development of the fetus, pregnant women, or women who might become pregnant, are advised not to take statins.

How Statins Work to Lower Cholesterol

Statins work by inhibiting an enzyme that is crucial to the manufacture of cholesterol by the body. (An enzyme is a specialized protein that helps to speed up a chemical reaction. For example, our digestive enzymes help speed up the breakdown of food into simple chemicals that can then be absorbed into the body.) Statins also increase the uptake of LDL cholesterol by the liver, another way in which they lower the blood level of cholesterol. The enzyme that is inhibited by statins works very early on in the synthetic pathway, (the synthetic pathway is like the assembly line in a factory; it is a set of chemical processes that occur inside cells as the body manufactures molecules it needs to survive). When this enzyme is inhibited the levels of other important molecules, such as coenzyme Q10 (more about that later), can also drop in people taking these medications.

Do I Need to Be on a Statin to Lower My Cholesterol?

So what should you do if your doctor informs you that you need to take a statin? The answer to whether or not you should follow that advice depends on your age, whether you are a man or a woman, and whether or not you have been diagnosed with atherosclerosis. Let me explain.

Atherosclerosis

Atherosclerosis is a form of hardening of the arteries in which plaque accumulates in the walls of arteries, eventually causing the opening of the vessels to narrow. When an artery becomes narrowed enough, the oxygen and nutrients carried by the blood cannot reach the organ supplied by that artery, starving it. For instance, the *coronary arteries* deliver blood to the heart. If the heart is not getting the amount of blood it needs—especially when it has to work harder, as it does during exercise or times of emotional stress—it is said to be *ischemic*. The term *ischemia* means a relative lack of blood supply. Hence, the terms *ischemic heart disease* (*IHD*), or *coronary heart disease* (*CHD*).

The symptom experienced by people whose hearts are being deprived of oxygen is called *angina pectoris*. Angina usually feels like a squeezing, burning, or pressure in the chest that is predictably brought on by exercise or emotional stress, and that goes away within about five minutes with rest, relaxation, or a medicine called nitroglycerin.

In addition to obstructing arteries to the point where blood flow is compromised, plaques can also rupture. A plaque that ruptures resembles an abscess or a boil in the wall of an artery. When the plaque material comes in contact with the blood flowing through that artery, the body tries to wall off this material by forming a blood clot (*thrombus*). If a clot forms over a ruptured plaque, blood flow through that artery can be completely interrupted, and the heart muscle downstream of the clot will die within a few hours if the circulation is not restored. Heart muscle damage from interruption of the blood supply is a *myocardial infarction*: a heart attack.

Risk Factors

We have a pretty good handle on the risk factors that make the development of atherosclerotic cardio-vascular disease (ASCVD) more likely. Only two of them can't be modified: your age and your family medical history. You can lie about your age, but, of course, that doesn't change it. And you might wish you had a different family and a different set of genes (I've always wanted to be taller), but we're more or less stuck with the genes we were born with. All the other risk factors—such as smoking, high blood pressure, abnormal levels of blood fats, diabetes, inflammation, being sedentary, and obesity—are modifiable, avoidable, or treatable.

Risk Factors for Developing Atherosclerosis	
CAN BE MODIFIED	CAN'T BE MODIFIED
Smoking	Age
Abnormal levels of cholesterol/triglycerides	Family history
High blood pressure	
Diabetes	
Obesity	
Sedentary life style	
Inflammation	

The more of those risk factors you have, the greater your chance of developing ASCVD. But the guidelines focus mostly on cholesterol levels. The current guidelines for the prevention of ASCVD state that the "optimal" level of total cholesterol is under 200, the "optimal" level of LDL cholesterol is under 100, and the "optimal" level of triglycerides is under 150. The latter was recently changed to under 100, although 150 is still given as the upper limit of normal. Note that these are "optimal" levels: they are not the levels that everyone needs to reach, especially since for many people, given their unhealthy diet and lifestyles, such levels are achievable only with drugs.

Table 1. Optimal Levels of Blood Fats	
Total cholesterol	Under 200
LDL cholesterol	Under 100
Triglycerides	Under 100

The guidelines that doctors are supposed to follow to prevent ASCVD say that your physician needs to determine the number of risk factors that you have, other than your LDL cholesterol level. Then, based on these, he or she classifies you as being at low, intermediate, or high risk. These other risk factors include age (forty-five years or older for men; fifty-five years or older for women), smoking, hypertension (blood pressure of 140/90 or more, or being on an antihypertensive medicine), low HDL cholesterol (under forty in a man, under fifty in a woman), and a family history of premature coronary heart disease in a male first-degree relative (father, brother, son) less than fifty-five years of age or in a female first-degree relative (mother, sister, daughter) less than sixty-five years of age. (For reasons we don't understand, women, even at equivalent levels of risk, tend to develop ASCVD ten to fifteen years later than men do.)

Table 2. Major Risk Factors (Other Than LDL Cholesterol) That Modify LDL Goals*

- Cigarette smoking
- High blood pressure
- Low HDL cholesterol (under 40 in men, under 50 in women)
- Family history of premature coronary heart disease
- Age (forty-five and over in men, fifty-five and over in women)

---

*   If HDL is 60 or more, this counts as a "negative" risk factor, and its presence allows you to subtract one risk factor from the total count. (Negative risk factor in this case means that high HDL cholesterol *lessens* the risk of developing plaque.)

For people who already have ASCVD or its equivalent (diabetes is considered a CHD risk equivalent), the "goal" should be to get the LDL cholesterol under 100. If someone has ASCVD and multiple other risk factors, then an *optional goal* is an LDL cholesterol under 70.

If a patient has zero to one risk factors—in other

words, someone at low risk—then the LDL cholesterol goal is under 160, and the guidelines state that drug therapy should be considered if the LDL cholesterol is 190 or greater.

If someone has two or more risk factors, the LDL cholesterol goal is under 130,* and if someone has established vascular disease or diabetes, the LDL cholesterol goal is under 100. The guidelines state that the first line of therapy in any case is therapeutic lifestyle changes—more on that later in chapter 5.

Table 3. Three Categories of Risk that Determine LDL Cholesterol Goals	
RISK CATEGORY	LDL GOAL
ASCVD and its equivalents	Under 100 (optional under 70)
2 or more risk factors	Under 130
0 to 1 risk factor	Under 160

---

*   If someone has two or more risk factors, physicians are urged to determine the absolute risk of a cardiac event over the next ten years using the Framingham risk score. The Framingham risk score takes into account age, total cholesterol, HDL cholesterol, smoking status, gender, and blood pressure. A Framingham risk score of 20 percent or more is considered an ASCVD risk equivalent. A risk score between 10 percent and 20 percent is considered intermediate risk and less than 10 percent is considered low risk. Low-risk people, even if they have two risk factors, have an LDL cholesterol goal of under 160, and drug therapy is advised if LDL cholesterol is 190 or more, while people at intermediate risk have an LDL cholesterol goal of under 130 and drug therapy should be considered if LDL cholesterol is above 160.

Unfortunately, many physicians don't read the complete set of guidelines. They read that the "optimal" LDL cholesterol goal is under 100, and willy-nilly they advise anyone with an LDL cholesterol over that number to go on a statin.

These guidelines are written by panels of prestigious medical scientists, many of whom have directed the clinical trials that produced the findings used to justify the recommendations in the guidelines. These trials have included tens of thousands of people from around the globe, and have compared drugs (usually statins) to placebos. Many of these researchers make significant amounts of money by conducting these trials, which are often sponsored by the pharmaceutical companies that make the drug being studied. These same researchers are often on the drug company's speakers bureaus and get paid handsomely for lecturing on the benefits of its products. The issue of conflict of interest bedevils medical science to a greater extent today than at any time in history.

Are the Guidelines Valid for Women?

There is another problem with the guidelines if you are a woman. The vast majority of the people who took part in the clinical trials that showed the benefit of lowering cholesterol were men. Some clinical trials excluded women, and others had only a small percentage of women participating. In many such trials, there were not enough female participants to determine if statin treatment had a beneficial effect in women.

It used to be thought that you could just take clinical trial results in men and apply them to women. But as more and more women have been studied, it's become apparent that women may benefit less than men may from certain medicines. Statins are in this category, but the guidelines don't take the lesser benefit in women into account.

Cardiac Events Despite Statins

And even the most ardent statin supporters have to concede that despite statin treatment, most men and women with ASCVD continue to suffer cardiac events and to die of their disease. They still have a very high residual risk, no matter how low their LDL cholesterol goes. In fact, the absolute risk of having a cardiac event in someone who takes a statin to lower their cholesterol, whether they have ASCVD or not, is only reduced by a few percentage points.

This may be because LDL cholesterol is not the whole story. In fact, most people with atherosclerosis do not have terribly high levels of LDL cholesterol. It's far more common for them to have a constellation of risk factors called the *metabolic syndrome*. There are five components of this syndrome, and if you have any three of them, you are given this diagnosis. The five are:

1. Abdominal or visceral obesity, defined as having a waist that measures more than forty inches if you are a man, and more than thirty-five inches if you are a women.

2. Elevated triglyceride level of 150 or more.
3. HDL cholesterol less than 40 in men and less than 50 in women.
4. Blood pressure of 130/85 or greater.
5. Fasting blood glucose (sugar) of 100 or more.

Since statins target mainly LDL cholesterol levels and have little effect on triglycerides or HDL cholesterol—in fact, high doses of statins usually *lower* the good cholesterol—there is still a high residual risk of atherosclerosis progressing in people taking the drugs, especially if they continue with unhealthy diets and lifestyles.

As you'll see in subsequent chapters, if you have established ASCVD, a statin will reduce your risk of having an event like a heart attack by a modest amount. If you are a woman with ASCVD, your risk will be reduced less than it will be in a man. If you are a man who has risk factors but hasn't been diagnosed with ASCVD, taking a statin to lower unhealthy levels of cholesterol will also lower your risk of future cardiac events by a small amount. But if you are a healthy woman, there is *zero* evidence that taking a statin will lower your risk of a heart attack or of dying of heart disease.

Based on the results of the JUPITER trial, the FDA has approved the expanded indication for rosuvastatin to include women ages sixty and older and men ages fifty and over who have normal levels of LDL cholesterol, increased inflammation based on an hsCRP blood test result of over 2, and one other risk factor. But I am seeing more and more healthy women in their thirties being put on this drug because their physicians don't read the fine print. A healthy woman in her thirties can expect to live another fifty years. It makes no sense at all to go on powerful medicines with the potential for serious, life-threatening side effects—for decades—when they have *no proven benefit*. Especially since you can get all of the benefits of statins without taking them, simply by changing your lifestyle.

Questions for Your Doctor

So what questions do you need to ask your physician if he/she wants you to take a statin?

1. Can I try altering my diet first to see if my cholesterol numbers improve? And if so, what diet should I follow?
2. Can you explain to me what my cholesterol numbers mean and how, according to the current guidelines, I meet the criteria for going on a statin?
3. Can you calculate my Framingham risk score and tell me what my risk is of having a cardiac event in the next ten years? (The National Institutes of Health has a website that allows you to figure out your own Framingham risk score, at www.nhlbi.nih.gov/guidelines/cholesterol/risk_tbl.htm#men.)
4. If diet doesn't get my cholesterol to a healthier level, could I take other, safer medicines than statins?

5. Is the dose of statin you are prescribing considered high, low, or average?

6. You say that my CRP is high and that even though my cholesterol is not elevated, I need to go on a statin. But I do not have any other risk factors, and I'm a fifty-year-old woman. Doesn't that mean I don't meet the criteria for being put on a statin?

It has never been more important to be an informed patient, asking questions of your physician and insisting on answers that you can understand. Armed with the information in this chapter, you will be better able to determine whether drug therapy to manage your cholesterol levels is really necessary. In the next chapter, I will go into greater detail about the "science" being used to justify the use of statins and the very real limitations of clinical trials.

Chapter 2

When Statins Help Most, and When They May Not Help at All

B.J. is a fifty-year-old teacher who developed sharp chest pain that traveled up to her neck and shoulders. It occurred off and on but was not worse while she was exerting herself. She went to her local hospital's emergency room and was admitted. B.J. underwent a nuclear stress test in which a radioactive tracer is used to detect areas of the heart that may not receive adequate blood flow during exercise. The results were normal. She had never been a smoker, was not diabetic, did not have high blood pressure, and was slightly overweight. Her parents were in their late seventies; both had high cholesterol but no heart disease. Her total cholesterol was 275, her triglycerides were 165, her HDL cholesterol was 53, and her LDL cholesterol was 189. She was started on simvastatin and developed diffuse pain in her muscles.

B.J. came to me for a second opinion, and I stopped the statin medicine and gave her extensive instruction on a seafood-vegetarian diet. Four months later, she was feeling well, her total cholesterol had come down to 238, her triglycerides had come down to 152, her HDL cholesterol had increased to 60, and her LDL cholesterol had come down to 148. Her goal according to current guidelines is an LDL cholesterol under 160.

———

T.C. was a sixty-two-year-old mechanic when he first came to see me in 1998. He had been diabetic for three years, and he was being treated with a fibrate medication for high triglyceride levels.(Fibrates are medicines that target triglycerides but have little effect on LDL cholesterol.) He had smoked three to four cigars per day until a year prior to seeing me, and he had a brother who'd suffered a heart attack in his early fifties. Over the three months prior to his visit, T.C. had developed shortness of breath and heaviness in his chest when he exerted himself. Despite taking his fibrate medicine, his triglyceride level was very elevated at 442. His total cholesterol was 159, and his HDL cholesterol was low at 27.

I sent him for a nuclear stress test. The result was very abnormal, and he underwent a heart catheterization, a diagnostic procedure in which specialized catheters are inserted into arteries and veins and advanced into the heart, enabling doctors to determine if there are obstructions in the arteries supplying the heart, the coronary arteries. The procedure showed extensive blockages in all the major branches of his coronary arteries. A statin medicine was added to his regimen. T.C. was felt not to be a good candidate for either bypass surgery or a balloon angioplasty/stent. (In a bypass operation, either another artery, or a vein is used to bypass a blockage in a coronary artery; in a balloon angioplasty, a specialized catheter with a balloon at its tip is advanced across an arterial narrowing and inflated to widen the artery. This area is then usually treated with a hollow mesh stent, to aid in keeping the artery open.) He did well for the next eight years but then developed increasing shortness of breath on exertion and fatigue. A repeat heart catheterization showed that the narrowing in his left coronary artery had increased. His numbers at that time were a total cholesterol of 147; triglycerides, 192; HDL, 30; and LDL, 79. T.C. received a stent and noticed improvement in his shortness of breath. Since that time (2006), he has done well.

———

These two patients represent the opposite ends of the spectrum for statin use. B.J. did not meet the current prevention guidelines for being put on a statin, she experienced almost immediate side effects, and diet alone was able to improve all of her levels. T.C., on the other hand, had every known risk factor, severe vascular disease, and very unhealthy blood-fat levels. He tolerated a low dose of statin medicine for many years and, despite his extensive coronary artery disease, has not had a heart attack. So how did we get to the point where two very different people were treated with the same class of medicine?

In this chapter, I will describe some of the studies that have compared statins to inactive placebo pills in an attempt to determine their risks and benefits. As with any venture that involves human beings, things are not as the claims of drug advertisements would have you believe.

Proving the "Cholesterol Hypothesis"

When the FDA approved the first statin drug, lovastatin (Mevacor), for sale in the United States in 1987, we had evidence that it was very effective at lowering LDL cholesterol, but no evidence that doing so would also reduce the risk of cardiovascular disease (CVD). In fact, the so-called cholesterol hypothesis was still quite controversial. Simply stated, the cholesterol hypothesis holds that abnormal cholesterol levels promote the buildup of plaque in arteries. In order to "prove" the cholesterol hypothesis, one would have to show that improving abnormal cholesterol levels decreased the amount of plaque accumulation.

In chapter 9, I will go into greater detail about the scientific method and the various clinical trials that have helped make statins the most widely prescribed drugs in the world. But for now, you just need to get a sense of how medical studies are carried out, what the reported results mean, and how errors can creep into even the best-designed trials. For the rest of this chapter, we'll be discussing trials in which a statin was compared to a placebo. The two groups of people enrolled in such studies are called the *intervention* group (those taking a statin) and the *control* group (those taking a placebo).

Primary and Secondary Prevention Trials

There are two types of clinical studies that are most pertinent to this discussion. A *primary prevention trial* seeks to show that in people *without evidence of CVD*, those treated with a statin will be less likely to have a heart attack or stroke or to die of heart disease over the course of the trial than those taking a placebo. A *secondary prevention trial* seeks to show that in people *with evidence of CVD*, those treated with a statin will suffer fewer subsequent events such as heart attack, stroke, or cardiac death over the course of the trial than those taking a placebo. These medical events are called *end points*, and clinical trial investigators follow the participants closely to determine if any of these end points occurs.

Primary Versus Secondary Prevention Trials

A primary prevention trial recruits people who *have no evidence* of a disease and treats them with either a drug or placebo to see if the drug prevents them from developing the disease. A secondary prevention trial recruits people who *have evidence* of a disease and treats them with either a drug or placebo to see if the drug lessens the likelihood of subsequent complications from the disease.

The best-designed clinical trials have "hard" end points such as heart attacks or death. (*Hard* in that they are end points with clear-cut definitions and are hard to miss—we docs don't often get death wrong.) But sometimes investigators include what are considered "soft" end points, like symptoms such as angina or the "need" for procedures like *angioplasty* (also called *percutaneous coronary intervention,* or *PCI), stents,* or coronary bypass surgery. The problem with these softer end points is that they are not really end points—they are decisions made by doctors taking care of people, and different physicians have very different thresholds for recommending these procedures.

For example, large clinical trials often involve people from many different countries. The JUPITER trial, which compared rosuvastatin (Crestor) to placebo in healthy people, took place in twenty-six countries, from the United States to Bulgaria. You don't have to be a genius to suspect that more bypass operations, stent placements, and angioplasties are performed in America than in Bulgaria. The results of these trials are said to be *statistically significant* if the likelihood is less than 5 percent that the difference in results between the intervention and the control groups could have occurred by chance. To be statistically significant, researchers calculate the *p value.* Most studies consider a statistically significant p value to be one that is less than 0.05, meaning there is less than a 5 percent likelihood that the results are due to chance.

Randomized, Placebo-Controlled, Double-Blind Trials

In the most scientifically valid studies, neither the people enrolled in the study nor the investigators running the clinical trial know which subjects are taking the active drug, a statin in the trials we'll be examining, and which are taking a placebo until after the study ends. This type of study is called a *randomized, placebo-controlled, double-blind trial.* This state of ignorance helps to avoid bias. For example, if an investigator knew that a certain subject in a clinical trial was taking a placebo, he or she might be more inclined to send that person for a stent or bypass, based on the knowledge that the people in the control group weren't receiving therapy. It is also important that the active drug group and the placebo group be as evenly matched for other risk factors as possible. In other words, you don't want to have 90 percent of the smokers in the placebo group and 10 percent of the smokers in the statin group, because smoking alone greatly increases the risk of heart attack, stroke, and death. So you want the people in the

---

* Clinical trials must be distinguished from other medical studies, like observational studies, in which individuals (for example, postmenopausal women taking hormone replacement pills) are observed over time and various outcomes (for example, the number of heart attacks or fractures) are measured and compared to a similar group of women not taking hormones. Observational studies are not experiments. No attempt is made to intervene with a drug or other therapy. And they are subject to what is called "selection bias." For example, postmenopausal women who chose to take hormone replacement medicines might also have been more likely to be of normal weight and not to smoke and therefore be at lower risk of heart disease than women who do not take postmenopausal hormones.

study to be very similar in all respects—except that one group is getting a real drug and the other group is getting a placebo. Once you have these two similar groups, you then assign them randomly to receive either active drug or placebo. The studies are planned to run for a set period of time; usually three to five years for statin trials.

All clinical trials nowadays have independent overseers, called data monitoring and safety boards, whose members do know who's getting what, and they meet periodically to go over the data from the study. If they determine that more people on the active drug are, say, having heart attacks and dying than the people on placebo, the study will be terminated prematurely. This happened with the highly touted Pfizer drug torcetrapib, a medication that raised levels of HDL cholesterol *and* lowered LDL cholesterol. The potential market for this drug was huge, and the pharmaceutical giant invested hundreds of millions of dollars in its development. In 2006 Pfizer CEO Jeff Kindler was quoted as saying, "This will be one of the most important compounds of our generation." Unfortunately, just days later, the preliminary results of a clinical trial comparing torcetrapib plus atorvastatin (Lipitor) to atorvastatin alone were made public: patients who received the drug combination had a 60 percent increase in mortality. That is to say they were 60 percent more likely to die than the subjects on Lipitor only. The study was scrapped immediately, as were several others investigating torcetrapib, and that spelled the end of Pfizer's miracle drug. The next day, Pfizer stock price tumbled 11 percent.

Reporting the Results of Clinical Trials

When the results of clinical trials are reported, the number of end points in the treated group is compared with the number of end points in the control group. This figure is often given as a percentage. Let's say, hypothetically, that the rate of the occurrence of an end point such as heart attack was 5 percent in the people given statins over the course of the study, and the rate of the occurrence of an end point was 10 percent in the people given the placebo. The *absolute risk reduction* is therefore 5 percent (10 percent minus 5 percent). But the *relative risk reduction* is a whopping *50 percent* (10 percent minus 5 percent divided by 10 percent). Guess which number gets touted when these clinical trials are reported?

Secondary Prevention with Statins

If we look at six of the secondary prevention trials of statins versus placebo (or in one case, high-dose statin compared to low-dose statin), the number of men in these trials totaled just over forty-one thousand, while the number of women totaled just under thirteen thousand. These studies lasted anywhere from three to six years. The results in men compared to women were different.

Close to 23 percent of the men on placebo had cardiac end points compared to almost 16 percent of men on statins. The absolute risk reduction was, therefore, a paltry 7 percent, although when you read about these trials, the authors always touted the relative risk reduction, which in this case was 30 percent.

But the women in these studies had different results. Just over 17 percent of women in the control group experienced cardiac events, compared to just under 13 percent of women in the statin-treated group. The absolute risk reduction for women in these studies was 4.5 percent, with a relative risk reduction of 26 percent. So women in the control group—even at similar cholesterol levels—were less likely to have an event than men were. Furthermore, the women who were assigned to statins saw their risk lowered less than the men did.

Primary Prevention with Statins

When you look at primary prevention trials, the results are even less impressive. I've analyzed the three out of four such studies that included women. In primary prevention trials, the participants do not have established atherosclerotic cardiovascular disease but are at increased risk of ASCVD. These three studies enrolled a total of 9,740 women and 24,972 men with an average age of fifty-eight to sixty-six. None of the clinical trials included people under the age of forty. Each study demonstrated a significant decrease in the occurrence of the primary end point in the study groups overall. The primary end point used in two of the trials was a composite of hard events like heart attack/cardiac death (or total deaths), and softer end points like the need for revascularization, or the need to be hospitalized for increasing chest pain, called unstable angina. Only one trial used the composite end point of either non-fatal heart attack or death from heart disease.

The absolute risk reductions in these three trials were a paltry 1 percent to 2 percent. (The overall event rates in these primary prevention trials were on the order of 2 percent to 5 percent, so much lower than the event rates in secondary prevention trials.) But the relative risk reductions were between 37 percent and 44 percent. Again, two of these trials included in their primary end points the softer end points of unstable angina or the need for revascularization (angioplasty, stent, or bypass surgery).

The results in women were even more underwhelming. If you look at the three studies' hard end points—nonfatal heart attack or cardiac death—40 women out of 4,904 on statins had either a heart attack or cardiac death, compared to 44 women out of 4,836 on placebo. Whether a woman took a statin or a placebo in these trials, her risk of suffering a heart attack or dying from her heart condition was less than 1 percent. This risk was 0.8 percent in women taking statins and 0.9 percent in women taking placebos, an absolute difference of 0.1 percent. This is *not* a significant statistical difference: over 1,000 women would have to take a statin to prevent one heart attack or cardiac death. Since the likelihood of experiencing a statin side effect is about 20 percent to 25 percent, the risk of putting a healthy

woman on a statin far outweighs the benefit. And yet
Big Pharma is trying very hard to obscure that fact with
intensive ad campaigns, directed at doctors and the
general public, touting the safety and efficacy of statins.

Why Clinical Trials Are Not All They're Cracked Up to Be

As I know from my own experience as a principal investigator, a lead researcher on a scientific investigation, clinical trials are not as cut-and-dried as we would
like to think. The data are analyzed by comparing the
treated group to the control group, using *intention to
treat*. This means that if you are in a clinical trial, and
you decide at some point that you want to stop taking
the drug being studied (even though you don't know
whether you are taking the active drug or the placebo),
you are perfectly within your rights to do so. However,
when the number of end points is totaled up at the end
of the study, you will be counted as being either in the
treatment group or the control group *even though you
weren't taking either*. Every clinical trial has such people, and they can influence the results for better or for
worse. In some clinical trials, as many as 50 percent of
the participants have discontinued the study drug by
the time the trial ends. They still get included in the
analysis, though. And then guidelines are promulgated
based on these clinical trial results, and doctors risk being accused of practicing substandard medicine if they
don't treat their patients as the guidelines suggest.

Another major problem with clinical trials is that

they are a very poor way to determine if the drug being studied is likely to produce serious side effects. All trials exclude many people who might be expected to take the drug once it has been approved by the FDA, or once the drug is promoted widely to doctors by sales representatives and to the general public by advertising. For example, these trials exclude the very elderly, people with liver or kidney disease, or those with any chronic illness that might "muddy" the results. In addition, they often won't accept patients taking other medicines—particularly other medicines that affect cholesterol levels. The usual duration of these trials is a few years, and sometimes side effects become apparent only after many years of use.

The Baycol Debacle

The story of cerivastatin (Baycol), a statin that was taken off the market in 2001, is instructive. Cerivastatin was manufactured by Bayer Pharmaceuticals. In previous clinical trials of other statins, anywhere from 0 percent to 0.5 percent of the participants reported muscle pain associated with a rise in the muscle enzymes that appear in the blood in cases of muscle damage. The most severe form of muscle damage, called *rhabdomyolysis*, occurred in only one trial in the 1990s and that involved a very high dose of a sustained-release form of simvastatin (Zocor), the third statin drug approved by the FDA.

When cerivastatin came to market in 1997, it was the most potent statin. The 0.4-milligram dose lowered cholesterol the same amount as 10 milligrams of another statin, Lipitor. Scientists at Bayer urged that the highest dose should be no more than 0.4 milligrams because "The safety margin for our compound from the no-effect level to nontolerable dose is less than three-fold, whereas for [Mevacor] it is at least 12-fold."[1] Despite this warning from its own scientists, Bayer sought and received permission to market a 0.8-milligram dose, even though company executives already knew that there were increasing reports of rhabdomyolysis in people taking cerivastatin.

In support of its effort to have cerivastatin approved, Bayer had submitted clinical trial data from over 2,800 patients, none of whom showed evidence of muscle damage based on blood tests. But once cerivastatin was approved and in wider use, it became apparent that it was far more likely than other statins to cause rhabdomyolysis, particularly if it was taken with gemfibrozil (Lopid), a fibrate medicine used to lower triglycerides. In June 2000, Bayer executives met to discuss this unfortunate spanner in the works. They proposed a package insert that would instruct patients that they should not take these two drugs concurrently. However, the company's director of medical research "mentioned that this leaflet should not be prepared before 12 July 2000 when a meeting is scheduled with the FDA to discuss labeling for the 0.8 mg tablet," because, as they were told by a consultant who had once worked for the FDA, "if the FDA is already tuned in to this, you may have some resistance about the higher dose." The next month, the FDA approved the 0.8 mg dose of cerivastatin, and the following month, Bayer submitted an application for that package insert warning patients not to take cerivastatin with gemfibrozil.

Between September 2000 and February 2001, eighteen cases of fatal cerivastatin-associated rhabdomyolysis were reported worldwide. The following month, a group of Bayer executives reviewed twelve reports of death in the United States since the beginning of 2001. In only one of these cases was cerivastatin taken with gemfibrozil: the others were mainly in people taking just the 0.8-milligram dose. This dose was then taken off the market in the United States and in Europe.

In August 2001 Bayer decided to discontinue cerivastatin altogether, and it shared this information first with its shareholders. Later on the same day, the FDA informed the American public about the withdrawal of cerivastatin. A media frenzy ensued. Bayer came in for heavy criticism for informing investors before regulatory agencies and physicians. The company was also censured for some of its marketing practices. In Germany, the largest circulation newspaper printed an article entitled, "Are Our Doctors Open to Bribes?," recounting Bayer's alleged paying for a luxury trip on the Orient-Express for physicians who prescribed cerivastatin for at least twenty-five patients.

The only happy campers in this debacle were the liability lawyers, who promptly invited anyone who had taken cerivastatin to consider making a claim. An estimated fifty law firms set up websites where people could find help determining if they had a case against Bayer. Perhaps worst of all for the pharmaceutical company, its share price dropped from 45 euros to 33 euros within a week. The final death toll from rhabdomyolysis due to cerivastatin is pegged at thirty-one, but this is probably an underestimate.

So, in summary, statins have been shown to lower the risk of cardiac events in people with established atherosclerosis. The benefit is modest, is less in women than in men, and, despite statin therapy, people with ASCVD still face a significant risk of heart disease even when their LDL cholesterol is brought to very low levels.

In people without established vascular disease, a recent analysis of primary prevention trials involving more than sixty-five thousand participants showed that statins did not cause any statistically significant decrease in the total mortality rate.[2] In healthy men, statins will cause about a 1 percent to 2 percent decrease in the risk of suffering a cardiac event. In women without vascular disease or its equivalent, statins will not lower the risk of cardiac events *at all*.

There is one exception to my disinclination to put healthy women or men on statins, and that is in the rare patient who has *familial hypercholesterolemia*. People who have one dose of the gene that causes this disease have LDL cholesterol levels in the range of 300 to 400 and most die prematurely of ASCVD. This is a rare disease, so there are no big clinical trials limited to people with this disorder. Nevertheless, their risk of ASCVD is so high that the benefit of putting them on statins almost certainly outweighs the risk, at least in people who can tolerate them without side effects.

Chapter 3

Common Side Effects of Statins: Cautionary Tales

C.F. is a successful businesswoman who lives in a large city in the northeastern United States. She had always been very healthy and led an active lifestyle, exercising several times a week. She was slightly overweight, didn't smoke, and didn't have high blood pressure or diabetes. Her mother had high blood pressure and high cholesterol, and died suddenly at the age of sixty-seven. Her father had suffered a heart attack at age sixty and died of heart disease ten years later.

When C.F. was in her early forties, her physician noted that her cholesterol was ranging between 200 and 230, and her LDL cholesterol, which had been in the range of 100 to 110, had crept up to 130. He put her on simvastatin (Zocor), 20 milligrams a day. About six months later, she began noticing severe panic attacks, which were treated first with the antidepressants sertraline (Zoloft) and then paroxetine (Paxil), but the attacks only got worse. She was working out with a trainer, doing aerobic exercise and weight training, but she began noticing progressive arm and leg weakness. C.F. told her *physician, who stopped the simvastatin and switched her to ezetimibe (Zetia), a nonstatin drug that blocks the absorption of cholesterol from the bowel. Her muscle pain improved, but her panic attacks did not. She was weaned off the paroxetine with her psychiatrist's approval. In 2008 the ezetimibe was discontinued, and her physician put her on atorvastatin (Lipitor). On this statin, she developed episodes of severe chest pressure, and her pulse rate would increase to very high levels of 180 to 200 beats per minute. C.F. also developed tremors, and her body temperature was very variable. Her muscle pain and weakness recurred and were so severe that she was unable to exercise or even to work.*

Her physician stopped the atorvastatin and tried rosuvastatin (Crestor). On this medicine, she developed severe exhaustion and pain in the muscles of her hands and chest. Again she was unable to exercise or work and spent most of her time lying on a couch. At that point, her physician stopped the rosuvastatin and tried lovastatin (Mevacor), but once again C.F. complained of severe panic attacks and severe arm and chest pain. She was also light-headed and weak. After two weeks on lovastatin, her physician tried fluvastatin (Lescol), but still her side effects remained the same. Finally, he tried pravastatin (Pravachol)—no improvement. So she stopped taking any statin medication, and gradually her symptoms all improved. After several months off statins, her HDL cholesterol was 55 and her LDL cholesterol was 130.

C.F. was concerned about the history of cardiovascular disease in both her parents, and an ultrasound of her carotid arteries (two large blood vessels in the neck that deliver blood to the brain) showed a minor degree of plaque. She wanted to bring down her cholesterol, so she asked her doctor about cholestyramine (Questran), which belongs to a family of drugs called bile acid sequestrants, and long-acting niacin (Niaspan—niacin is a B vitamin that in high doses raises HDL cholesterol, lowers LDL cholesterol and lowers triglycerides). She was started on these medications and felt fine. She continues on them to this day. C.F. has enough energy to work at her demanding job, runs regularly for exercise, and is no longer crippled by anxiety attacks. Her total cholesterol varies between 160 and 190, her HDL cholesterol is 90, and her LDL cholesterol is 80.

———

A.G. is an attorney who practices in the southern United States. He had no family history of coronary heart disease, was not diabetic, had never smoked, and did not have high blood pressure. He was overweight but had no symptoms of heart disease. His primary care doctor had referred him to a cardiologist in 2006, when it was thought that he might have pericarditis (an inflammation in the sac around the heart), but this diagnosis was never confirmed, and his symptoms, which came on during an upper respiratory infection, went away completely.

He had been noted to have slightly elevated cholesterol levels for about eight years. In November 2007 A.G.'s total cholesterol was 213, his LDL cholesterol was 135, his HDL cholesterol was 44, and his triglycerides were 173. At that point, his cardiologist suggested that he start Vytorin, a combination of simvastatin and ezetimibe. In his office note, the cardiologist said that National Cholesterol Education Program (NCEP) guidelines "would suggest LDL less than 100, HDL greater than 45, triglycerides less than 150, and total cholesterol less than 200."

But the physician was in error: the LDL of less than 100 refers to people with established atherosclerotic cardiovascular disease (ASCVD), or those with an absolute risk of developing this disease of more than 20 percent over the next ten years. In fact, A.G. did not have established ASCVD, and his ten-year Framingham risk score was calculated at 7 percent. According to current guidelines, there was no reason to put him on statins.

A.G. refused to take a statin at that time, but a year later, when his cholesterol was checked again, the total had gone up to 239, the LDL was 150, the HDL was 46, and the triglycerides were 214. At that point, the cardiologist prescribed 40 milligrams of simvastatin (a fairly high dose) and fish oil tablets, which can lower triglycerides when taken in high doses. On January 16, 2009, A.G. took the first dose of simvastatin the night before flying to Las Vegas on vacation. Within twenty-four hours, he developed back pain and difficulty walking, which he at first attributed to his having carried a heavy suitcase and some residual pain from a car accident he'd been in a month before. Later in the week, however, A.G.'s thigh became so tight that no amount of stretching or massage would make it better, and his urine had become very dark in color. He began having diffuse muscle spasms. He was also having difficulty concentrating and understanding conversations going on around him. On the plane ride home, he felt extremely ill, with a severe headache. He thought he might be coming down with the flu and stayed home from work for the next week.

A few weeks later, he resumed working out with his personal trainer, whom he'd known for two years. As A.G. recounted in an email message, "He had commented in early January that I was training as hard as a Navy SEAL . . . or at least I felt like I could keep up with Navy SEALs.

"After one exercise, he looked at me and asked me why I was so weak. He couldn't believe how weak I was. I told him I thought I was getting over the flu, but he told me it was much worse than that. (He set the weights I was to lift, and he had put on only warm-up weights, and I couldn't get through those.) He tried one more very light exercise, and my lower back went out on me. We stopped just minutes into the routine, and I then began to realize something was wrong."

On his own, A.G. began reading up on statin side effects. He stopped the simvastatin, even though the nurse at his doctor's office suggested that he just cut down on the dose. But he continued to have multiple symptoms, including facial pain and twitching, hand pain, neck pain, upper and lower back pain, and difficulty concentrating. He went to a pain center, where an electroneuromyogram (EMG—a test that measures the electrical activity of muscle tissue) was abnormal, revealing problems with nerve conduction in both of his legs. Next he went to a world-renowned center, which did another EMG; again it was abnormal, in both the upper and lower extremities. In his own words:

> I am an attorney and still searching for ways to get better. However, sixteen doses of that 40 milligrams of simvastatin have ruined my health and my career. I have cognitive difficulties that relate back to that first week in Vegas when I was missing entire conversations. In addition, I have continuous muscle pain and twitching, as my entire neuromuscular system has been affected. I have been evaluated by many doctors, but no one so far has been able to truly help me.
>
> As an attorney, I am trying to expend what little energy I have to researching these drugs and informing others to be careful. I think the secret is in the dosage as it relates to the cholesterol levels of people.
>
> I want justice for myself and all the other victims, but many lawyers have a hard time understanding how to put the case together, especially with so many cardiologists singing the praises of statin drugs and ignoring those patients who complain of serious side effects. (I have yet to receive a phone call from my doctor after I phoned his office to tell him I was stopping the medication because of the side effects. He didn't report the side effects to the FDA, and he didn't even note my phone call in the chart.)

Interestingly, A.G.'s mother had experienced a bad reaction to statins also. To this day, more than two years later, he continues to suffer from pain, muscle twitching, cognitive issues, which interfere with his ability to function as an attorney, and chronic fatigue.

———

L.M. is a cardiothoracic surgeon at a university medical center. His cardiologist put him on lovastatin for slightly elevated cholesterol levels. After about six months, when there was no drop in his levels, the dose was doubled. Shortly thereafter, he awoke one morning with burning pain and loss of sensation in his left foot. Convinced that he had developed a clot in his leg, L.M. examined himself. But the pulse in his foot was fine, and there was no bluish discoloration of the skin, as would occur if blood flow to the foot were compromised. Tests showed normal circulation to the feet.

After about a week, the pain spread to involve his whole lower leg. The pain was so severe that for the first time in his life, L.M. took Percocet, a strong pain medicine that contains the narcotic oxycodone plus acetaminophen. Then he developed pain over the rib cage in his lower chest. He saw two neurologists, who told him that he had shingles and put him on medication. But he never developed the characteristic blistered skin rash, and blood tests failed to show any evidence of shingles. The pain lasted for several months. Finally, L.M. took himself off lovastatin, and the pain went away within a matter of days. He hasn't taken a statin since.

The immediate impetus for my writing this book was the news that the FDA had approved the expanded indication for statin use in healthy people with normal cholesterol levels, based on the flawed JUPITER study. But even before that, I had become more and more concerned about patients—my own and others that I'd read of or learned about—who were experiencing serious side effects to statin medicines. For more than twenty years now, physicians have been assured over and over again that statins are safe—so safe that some enthusiasts suggested they could be put in the water supply. Others advise that everyone over the age of fifty-five should take a "polypill" containing aspirin, a blood pressure medication, and a statin. While we accept a significant chance of adverse effects when medicines are given to treat deathly ill people who might die, we need to have a lower tolerance for side

---

FDA Approved Statins

Fluvastatin (Lescol)

Simvastatin (Zocor)

Atorvastatin (Lipitor)

Lovastatin (Mevacor)

Pravastatin (Pravachol)

Rosuvastatin (Crestor)

---

effects if we are treating healthy people to bring about a small reduction in the risk of some future event that is unlikely to occur for many years. In the latter case, we need to be *very* sure that the benefits outweigh the risks. Especially when lifestyle changes that carry *no* risk can accomplish the same result. What follows is a summary of statin side effects that have been reported from around the world.

The Yin and Yang of Statins

Statin medicines are classic examples of entities that have positive and negative aspects. The positive aspects of statins include their ability to lower LDL cholesterol, to combat inflammation, to improve the function of the inner lining of arteries, to combat oxidation (the oxidized form of LDL cholesterol injures arteries, initiating the buildup of plaque), and to decrease the tendency of clots to form. Some scientists believe that the anti-inflammatory and antioxidant properties of statins are at least as important as their ability to lower LDL cholesterol. The end result of statin therapy is that plaque formation is inhibited (but not stopped), and any plaque that does form is less likely to rupture. (It is plaque rupture, with resultant clot formation, that causes most heart attacks.) The statins currently available in the United States are fluvastatin (Lescol), simvastatin (Zocor), atorvastatin (Lipitor), lovastatin (Mevacor), pravastatin (Pravachol), and rosuvastatin (Crestor).

Physicians are urged to practice "evidence-based medicine," and various august advisory panels promulgate guidelines based on the evidence gleaned from clinical trials. Physicians ignore these clinical practice guidelines at their own risk, especially in the litigious United States. For example, as was noted in chapter 1, current guidelines stipulate that anyone with diagnosed atherosclerotic cardiovascular disease and multiple risk factors should be treated, preferably with statins, to lower his or her LDL cholesterol below 100 and preferably below 70. Failing to do so, particularly if a patient does poorly, leaves the doctor vulnerable to a charge of malpractice for failure to abide by "accepted standards of practice." So the vast majority of physicians, myself included, prescribe statins for their at-risk patients, particularly those with ASCVD, or in those at high risk of ASCVD when lifestyle modification does not bring down LDL cholesterol to target levels. And many of these people tolerate statins quite well.

But statins have a dark side. Because they inhibit the action of *HMG-CoA reductase,* an enzyme early in the pathway leading to cholesterol synthesis, they also reduce other end products of this pathway, including *coenzyme Q10* (CoQ10). Sometimes called *ubiquinone,* CoQ10 is necessary for the proper functioning of cells and participates in the generation of cellular energy from little energy factories in our cells called *mitochondria.* About half of our CoQ10 comes from the fat in our diets, and the rest is manufactured within our bodies.

Statins can reduce blood levels of CoQ10 by 16 percent to 54 percent.[1] There are several diseases caused by malfunctioning mitochondria. These diseases may be inherited genetically or may be acquired—that is, they may develop sometime after birth. When mitochondrial dysfunction causes muscle damage, this is referred to as *mitochondrial myopathy*. Mitochondrial function declines as we age. Some investigators have reported evidence of mitochondrial dysfunction during statin treatment. Mitochondria are absolutely essential for survival, so defects in how our mitochondria function can have disastrous consequences.

Nerve cells, heart muscle cells, and skeletal muscle cells are particularly rich in mitochondria. These tiny energy producers contain their own DNA (genetic material called mtDNA), but, interestingly, unlike other cells, all of the DNA in our mitochondria comes from our mothers and none from our fathers.

The genetics of mtDNA are still being worked out, but it is clear that mitochondrial defects underlie several devastating diseases associated with deafness, blindness, diabetes, epilepsy, strokes, mental retardation, psychiatric illness, *myopathy* (abnormality or degeneration of muscles), neuropathy (abnormality or degeneration of nerves), and death. A few diseases caused by mitochondrial dysfunction have responded to treatment with CoQ10, and this is an area that is being investigated actively.

Rare associations between mutations in mtDNA have also been reported for some cases of Alzheimer's disease, Parkinson's disease, and amyotrophic lateral sclerosis, better known as Lou Gehrig's disease.

So, to reiterate, CoQ10 is vital to the normal functioning of mitochondria, and, as noted above, blood levels of CoQ10 are diminished by taking statins.

Muscle Side Effects of Statins

The most common side effect of statins, myopathy, occurs with increasing frequency the higher the dose and causes symptoms ranging from mild *myalgia* (muscle pain), cramps, tenderness, and weakness to the rare but life-threatening condition called rhabdomyolysis. This disorder causes severe damage to muscles all over the body. Muscle fibers die and release a protein called *myoglobin* into the bloodstream. Myoglobin is excreted by the kidney, and high blood levels can plug up the kidney's tubules and lead to kidney failure. The urine often turns a dark, almost mahogany color from the large amounts of myoglobin in the urine.

Rhabdomyolysis is sometimes fatal. The risk of rhabdomyolysis in people taking statins increases if they are also taking a wide range of other medicines, including other types of cholesterol-reducing agents called fibrates, some of the medicines used to treat AIDS, certain immunosuppressive drugs used in transplant patients to prevent rejection, and certain antibiotics, including some used to treat fungal infections. The risk of rhabdomyolysis is also increased in women, the elderly, those with uncontrolled infections or seizures, and people with kidney disease.

To emphasize a very important point, the risk increases when people are treated with higher doses of statins. On June 8, 2011, the FDA took note of this fact when it issued warnings on the use of high-dose simvastatin. In a letter to health care professionals, the FDA restricted the 80-milligram dose of simvastatin to those people who had been taking it for twelve or more months without evidence of what it called "muscle toxicity." The agency advised that the simvastatin 80-milligram dose, compared to other statins with similar or greater ability to lower LDL cholesterol, had an increased risk of muscle injury, including rhabdomyolysis. It also recommended that simvastatin not be used with many other medications, including certain antibiotics and drugs used to treat HIV/AIDS, and restricted the dose of simvastatin in people taking commonly prescribed medicines used to treat high blood pressure and angina.

As the goals for optimal LDL cholesterol are constantly revised downward, we can expect physicians to push their patients to take higher doses of statins. And the result may be more harm than good.

Revised FDA Prescribing Information on Simvastatin		
INTERACTING DRUG	PREVIOUS LABEL	UPDATED LABEL
Antifungals		
itraconazole (Sporanox)	Avoid	Contraindicated
ketoconazole (Feoris, Nizoral)		
posaconazole (Noxafil)		
HIV Protease Inhibitors		
saquinavir, ritonavir, indinavir, others	Avoid	Contraindicated
Antibiotics		
erythromycin (goes by several brand names)	Avoid	Contraindicated
clarithromycin (Biaxin)		
telithromycin (Ketek)		
Antidepressants		
nefazodone (Serzone)	Avoid	Contraindicated
Fibrates		
gemfibrozil (Gemcor, Lopid)	Do not exceed 10 milligrams of simvastatin daily	Contraindicated
Immunosuppressants		
cyclosporine (goes by several brand names)	Do not exceed 10 milligrams of simvastatin daily	Contraindicated

Synthetic Steroids		
danazol (Danocrine)	Do not exceed 10 milligrams of simvastatin daily	Contraindicated

Other medicines should not be administered with certain doses of simvastatin. These are:		
INTERACTING DRUG	PREVIOUS LABEL	UPDATED LABEL
Antiarrhythmics		
amiodarone (Cordarone, Pacerone)	Do not exceed 20 milligrams daily	Do not exceed 10 milligrams daily
Calcium Channel Blockers		
verapamil (goes by several brand names)	Do not exceed 20 milligrams daily	Do not exceed 10 milligrams daily
diltiazem (goes by several brand names)	Do not exceed 40 milligrams daily	Do not exceed 10 milligrams daily
amlodipine (Norvasc)	No dose cap	Do not exceed 20 milligrams daily
Antianginals		
ranolazine (Ranexa)	No dose cap	Do not exceed 20 milligrams daily

Although rhabdomyolysis is rare, it is common for people taking a statin to complain of muscle pain and weakness. While most medical literature says that this occurs in about 10 percent of people taking statins, in my experience, the incidence is more like 20 percent. This is in line with the findings of a French study which found that among 815 people treated with lipid-lowering drugs, 23 percent experienced muscle symptoms.[2] These appeared soon after the medicine was started and went away when the drug was discontinued.

The cause of statin myopathy is not known, but there is reason to believe it might be related to low levels of CoQ10. The evidence that statin myopathy may be successfully treated with CoQ10 is not strong; the few small studies yield conflicting results. However, this area is under active investigation.

One of the best-known scientists looking closely at muscle function in people taking statins is Dr. Paul Thompson, the chief of cardiology at Hartford Hospital in Hartford, Connecticut. He is also director of Preventive Cardiology and of the Athletes' Heart programs there, and is a professor of medicine at the University of Connecticut. (A disclaimer: Dr. Thompson and I have been friends for years and were colleagues at one of the Brown University teaching hospitals in the 1980s.)

He currently has grants from the National Institutes of Health (NIH—the US government's medical research agency that supports medical research into many diseases) to study the effect of treatment with CoQ10 on statin myopathy, to study the effect of statins on skeletal muscle strength and performance, and to study the effects of statins on brain function.

In the CoQ10 study, he is recruiting 135 people who have developed muscle pain while taking statins. They will be treated in a double-blind fashion with either CoQ10 or placebo. At the completion of the study, we should have a better idea as to whether or not the estimated $400 million spent on CoQ10 treatment in the United States in 2008 was money well spent or money down the drain.

Despite the fact that so many people taking statins complain of muscle pain, muscle performance in these people has not received a lot of attention. Nowadays, when so much clinical research is paid for by Big Pharma, it is not surprising that no statin manufacturer has investigated the performance of various muscle groups in statin users.

But the NIH, which used to be the main sponsor of medical research in the United States, has seen fit to fund the research that may give us great insight into the actions of statins on muscles. Dr. Thompson's research will clarify what metabolic pathways are involved in statin muscle injury, and may ultimately help in the development of cholesterol-lowering medicines that don't injure muscles.

When someone on statins complains of muscle pain, the doctor often orders a *creatine phosphokinase* (*CPK*) test for muscle damage. CPK is an enzyme that is released into the blood when muscle cells are damaged. If the CPK level is more than ten times the upper limit of normal, that person is diagnosed with *myositis*, or muscle inflammation/damage, and the statin is discontinued.

But even if the CPK is not elevated, this does not mean that there is no muscle damage and that the statin is not causing the muscle pain. In 2002 a study found that four patients who reproducibly developed muscle pain on statins, but not placebo, had muscle biopsies that showed evidence of mitochondrial dysfunction. (A biopsy is a procedure in which a sample of tissue is removed from the body for examination and testing.) All had normal levels of CPK. Three of them agreed to be biopsied after they were off statins, and the abnormalities that were seen during statin therapy were no longer present. In addition, strength testing in these patients demonstrated muscle weakness on statins, which normalized on placebo.[3]

Unfortunately, all too often when patients on statins complain of muscle pain and the CPK test comes back normal, their doctor tells them that the statin is not responsible for their pain. Luckily, many people have enough sense to go off the statin, and most find their symptoms vastly improved within a few days.

Statins May Unmask Previously Undiagnosed Conditions

There are increasing reports in the medical literature of statin therapy unmasking previously unknown conditions such as McArdle's disease. People affected with McArdle's develop muscle pain and weakness after exercise. Statins have also been implicated in uncovering the presence of myotonic dystrophy, adult-onset muscular dystrophy, and in making people with the disease myasthenia gravis worse. In some people, the presence of myotonic dystrophy was only discovered when they developed muscle pain and weakness after being put on a statin. Lastly, statins have either unmasked or induced mitochondrial myopathies in people with previously undiagnosed mitochondrial defects.

More on Rhabdomyolysis and the Failure of RCTs to Detect It

Rhabdomyolysis is the most feared muscle side effect of statin use. A meta-analysis of randomized, controlled trials (RCTs) did not show a statistically increased risk of rhabdomyolysis in people on statins compared to placebo. (A meta-analysis combines the results of many studies.) However, RCTs may not succeed in finding evidence of increased risk of side effects, even when they do, in fact, exist. This is probably because most clinical trials last only a few years, and some side effects appear only after prolonged use.

Another way to look at drug effects is the *number needed to treat*, or *NNT*. This number tells physicians the number of people they need to treat to see an effect, whether beneficial or harmful. In a 2004 study, the NNT to see one case of rhabdomyolysis was only 9.7 to 12.7 for people taking the cerivastatin (Baycol)-fibrate combination, versus an NNT of 22,727 to see one case of rhabdomyolysis for those taking a statin other than cerivastatin alone.[4]

But rhabdomyolysis can occur with any statin. In one study, the side effect occurred one year after patients began the drug, on average; however, an unusual instance of rhabdomyolysis occurring after just one dose of a statin has been reported.[5] Others have reported rhabdomyolysis occurring two to four days after statin therapy was initiated. And while most people with rhabdomyolysis complain of diffuse, severe muscle pain and weakness, others may have a more insidious course, presenting with what sounds like the flu, or just fatigue, or low back pain, or shortness of breath.

Although rhabdomyolysis affects primarily muscles, it can lead to kidney failure and can cause toxic effects in heart muscle, the brain, the pancreas, the liver, the lung, and the bone marrow.

Interactions of Juices and Statins

In addition to the increased risk of adverse events (AEs) seen in people taking certain other medicines along with statins, grapefruit juice and pomegranate juice also increase the risk of muscle AEs. This is thought to occur because, much like the drugs that increase the risk of statin AEs, these juices inhibit enzymes that metabolize (break down) statins. This leads to higher blood levels of statins, which, as with increasing the dose of statins, increases the likelihood of side effects.

In 2006 an article by Dr. Paul Thompson and his colleagues reported on a patient who started drinking pomegranate juice while taking rosuvastatin and a blocker of cholesterol absorption from the bowel, ezetimibe.[6] This forty-eight-year-old man had been taking the drug combination for seventeen months without a problem. Then he began to drink less than a cup of pomegranate juice twice a week, because he'd read a report on its health benefits. Within three weeks, he developed muscle pain and was found to have a markedly elevated CPK level. Luckily, when his medicines and pomegranate juice were discontinued, the rhabdomyolysis resolved, and he made a full recovery. While some physicians caution their patients about drinking more than a quart of grapefruit juice a day, smaller quantities can also pose a risk. In a 1998 study, less than a cup of grapefruit juice a day drunk before the subjects took their simvastatin dose caused a nine-fold increase in peak simvastatin blood levels.[7] Again, this increase in statin blood levels occurs because grapefruits and pomegranates contain substances that interfere with the enzymes that normally metabolize statins in the body.

Statin-Induced Tendon Damage

Muscles are not the only parts of the musculoskeletal system that statins can affect. Tendons attach our muscles to our bones, and *tendonitis* (inflamed tendons) and even tendon rupture have been associated with statin therapy. New Zealand researchers published a study in which they searched the database of the World Health Organization (WHO). They found 205 cases of tendonitis, tendon disorder, or tendon rupture associated with statin use.[8]

A 2008 French study in the journal *Arthritis Care and Research* reported on tendon problems in 2 percent of 4,597 people, with side effects thought to be caused by statins.[9] These effects usually occurred within eight months of starting therapy. Most had tendonitis— primarily of the Achilles tendon in the back of the ankle but some suffered tendon rupture. Seventeen people had such severe symptoms that they needed to be hospitalized. In 2009 the *Journal of Cardiovascular Pharmacology* published a *case-control study* of statin use and tendon rupture.[10] A case-control study compares people who have a disease or condition (cases) with a group of people free of the disease or condition (controls) looking for factors that might increase the likelihood of disease. The authors looked at electronic medical records at Michigan State University from 2002 to 2007. They compared statin exposure in 93 people who had tendon rupture to 279 sex- and age-matched controls without tendon rupture. They found that women taking statins had an almost fourfold increased risk of tendon rupture compared to women not taking statins, but that men did not have an increased risk. Their conclusion was that statin use is a significant risk factor for tendon rupture in women but not in men.

Joint Problems with Statin Use

A Japanese study reported in 2001 on the association of shoulder stiffness with statin use.[11] The people in this study were taking lower doses of pravastatin (5 to 20 milligrams a day) or simvastatin (5 to 10 milligrams a day) than are commonly prescribed today. The researchers found that fourteen out of forty-three men (27 percent) and thirty-eight out of sixty-six women (58 percent) complained of shoulder stiffness while taking statins. Once again, women seem to be at a greater risk of statin complications.

Other patients (and I've seen this quite commonly in my own practice) complain of joint pain that appears while they are taking a statin and then goes away when they stop the drug. Of interest in this regard, a 2005 report in the *Journal of Rheumatology* found that statin use in women sixty-five years of age or older led to almost double the risk of developing osteoarthritis, or "wear and tear" arthritis of the hip.[12]

Statin Effects on the Liver

Abnormalities of liver function, discovered by way of a simple blood test, also can be caused by statins, and this AE is more apt to occur with increasing doses, the likelihood almost tripling when high-dose statins are compared to low-dose statins. That is why your physician checks your liver enzymes about every six months when you are taking a statin. Overall, 0.5 percent to 3 percent of people taking statins will have abnormal liver function tests. If the liver enzymes are increased more than three times the upper limit of normal, the statin should be stopped. Usually the abnormal liver blood test returns to normal after the statin has been discontinued, but not always.

In 2003 the *Journal of Hepatology* reported a fatal case of liver failure caused by atorvastatin in an eighty-three-year-old man.[13] The authors then reviewed the Adverse Event Reporting System of the World Health Organization for deaths resulting from serious liver injury clearly attributable to statin therapy. They found that fatal liver failure is rare among statin users, with reported rates less than one death per one million statin prescriptions. Of those with fatal liver injury, the age range was twenty to eighty-eight years, with a median age of sixty-four, and men and women were affected equally. (*Median* means that half were above this age and half were below.) However, since more men than women are prescribed statins, the authors raised the possibility that women might be more susceptible than men to serious liver injury from statins. And given that about forty million people in the United States take statins each year, we might be looking at dozens of cases of fatal liver injury.

Acute hepatitis (liver damage/inflammation which can have many different causes) was also reported in a woman taking a "natural" lipid-lowering product, which contained, in addition to other things, *red rice yeast*.[14] The reason that red rice yeast lowers cholesterol is that it contains lovastatin. The patient, an Italian woman, had previously exhibited elevated liver enzymes when she was prescribed lovastatin; her liver enzyme level returned to normal when the drug was discontinued. Despite this, another consultant prescribed over-the-counter Equisterol, which the manufacturer claims contains several ingredients, including niacin, CoQ10, and the plant-derived substances guggulsterol, and policosanol, in addition to red rice yeast. Viral hepatitis was ruled out by blood tests, as were other causes of hepatitis. In this case, the liver damage (confirmed by a liver biopsy) resolved when the supplement was stopped. Because statins can cause liver injury, they should not be taken by people who drink to excess or by those with known liver disease.

Statin Effects on Nerves and the Brain

Of all the reported statin side effects, the ones that worry me most are those that involve damage to nerves and the brain. A short digression here:

The nervous system is divided into the *central nervous system (CNS)*, made up of the brain and the spinal cord, and the *peripheral nervous system (PNS)*, composed of the nerves outside the central nervous system. The PNS is also divided into two parts: the *somatic nervous system*, which supplies nerves to our skin, muscles, and joints; and the *visceral nervous system*, also called the *autonomic nervous system (ANS)*, which provides nerves to our internal organs, blood vessels, and the glands that manufacture hormones. The CNS and the PNS are not really separate, as the spinal cord conducts information from both divisions of the PNS to the brain, while the brain also receives input from its own *cranial nerves*, which are involved with functions such as vision, smell, hearing, and taste. The brain processes all these inputs and then, for example, instructs a muscle to contract, or a gland to secrete a hormone, or the heart to speed up. So the CNS and PNS are in constant communication and influence each other.

Nerves are made up of bundles of *neurons,* complex cells that have slender projections called *dendrites* and *axons.* Dendrites, branching threadlike structures, allow the neuron to make connections to adjacent nerve cells. Nerves convey information in the form of electrochemical impulses. The dendrites detect these signals, which then travel along the axon and are transmitted to a neighboring cell across a small gap called the *synapse.*

Axons are enclosed in a protective layer of insulation called the *myelin sheath,* of which cholesterol is a key component. Myelin not only protects the axon from injury but also insulates the electrical impulses (just as electrical wires have rubber insulation to keep the electricity from leaking out and damaging nearby structures) and increases the speed at which they are transmitted—up to four hundred feet per second, in some cases.

Many human diseases are characterized by a loss of myelin, called *demyelination,* or by defective myelination, called *dysmyelination.* Examples of the former include multiple sclerosis and Guillain-Barre syndrome. Dysmyelination is thought to contribute to rare diseases including Canavan disease and phenylketonuria.

Next to muscle-related adverse effects, the next most common AEs reported by people taking statins involve cognitive impairment: interference with our ability to think, concentrate, remember, and solve mental problems. We know that mitochondrial density is high in brain tissue, we know that CoQ10 is necessary for normal mitochondrial function, and we know that statin therapy decreases CoQ10 levels. It's not surprising, therefore, that cognitive impairment is reported in people taking statins. In fact, there are inherited diseases characterized by CoQ10 deficiency in which the dominant symptoms are cognitive problems, including mental retardation, along with muscle symptoms, and gait abnormalities. An example is familial mitochondrial encephalopathy.

The effect of lovastatin on cognitive function was studied in a randomized, double-blind fashion by Dr. Matthew Muldoon and his colleagues at the University of Pittsburgh.[15] They recruited 209 healthy adults ages twenty-four to sixty with high levels of LDL cholesterol and randomly assigned them to either 20 milligrams of lovastatin or placebo daily. The volunteers were given standardized tests of neuropsychological performance at baseline—that is, before any treatment, and again at the end of the treatment period. They also filled out questionnaires on depression, anxiety, hostility, and quality of life. The people who took the placebo improved on all measures of neuropsychological performance between baseline and six months, as would be expected because of the effects of practice on test performance. Attention, psychomotor speed, (the amount of time someone takes to process information, prepare a response, and execute that response), mental flexibility, working memory, and memory recall all improved in the placebo group. Those treated with lovastatin improved only on tests of memory recall, and there were small but statistically significant declines in tests of attention and psychomotor speed. Psychological well-being was not affected by lovastatin.

In a later study, published in 2004, Dr. Muldoon and his colleagues looked at the effects of low-dose simvastatin (10 milligrams daily) or higher-dose simvastatin (40 milligrams daily) on cognitive function in 283 people with high levels of cholesterol.[16] The participants were randomly assigned to placebo or to one of the two statin doses and took a neuropsychological test battery at baseline and again at the end of six months. The authors concluded that the trial found only minor decreases in cognitive functioning with statins, and that the higher dose of simvastatin had no greater effects on cognitive performance than the lower dose. Both of these studies were of short duration, however, so it is conceivable that greater effects would have been seen if they were longer than just six months.

Dr. Paul Thompson became interested in the question of whether statins affect the brain because of a patient who developed difficulty with memory after being put on a statin. He has begun a study to examine brain function in people taking high-dose statins— in this case, 80 milligrams of atorvastatin daily, the maximum recommended dose. He has received funding from the NIH for this study. He will look at actual brain function using an imaging procedure called *functional magnetic resonance imaging* (*fMRI*), which makes it possible to observe metabolic activity in the brain in real time. The fMRI allows the doctor to view activation of the neurons in the brain in response to various tasks. The subjects will undergo fMRI tests while performing two different memory-based exercises during the high-dose atorvastatin therapy and while taking placebo. This will be done in a double-blind fashion. The subjects will also be administered standardized tests of cognitive function while on statins and while on placebo.

The study is still in its early stages, but according to preliminary findings, men and women on statins don't encode memory as efficiently as they do while on placebo, and they require more areas of the brain to perform mental tests. If these early observations are borne out, they will provide an explanation for the "brain fog" that some people experience when treated with statins.

Statin-Induced Nerve Damage

Peripheral nerves may also be affected by statin therapy. *Neuropathy* is the term that physicians use to describe damage to peripheral nerves. *Polyneuropathy* describes damage to multiple nerves. Nerve damage can be caused by diseases such as diabetes and shingles, by drugs, by genetic defects, and by exposure to certain toxins like pesticides and heavy metals. People with neuropathy can suffer debilitating pain, often in the feet and hands, or can have altered perception of pain, which can result in injury. They may experience *paresthesias*: abnormal sensations such as tingling, numbness, burning, or "pins and needles." Unfortunately, we do not have good treatments for neuropathy unless we can identify a specific cause and remove the offending agent.

Danish researchers published a report on their study of the risk of polyneuropathy in people on statins in 2002.[17] They used a population-based patient registry (registries identify and track certain diseases or conditions in a defined population) to determine how many cases of *idiopathic* (that is, of unknown cause) polyneuropathy were registered over a five-year period. They then randomly selected twenty-five times as many control subjects without polyneuropathy who were matched for sex and age. They used a prescription register to assess exposure to drugs and estimated the *odds ratio* of statin use in people with polyneuropathy compared to controls.

The odds ratio is a relative measure of risk. It tells us, for example, how likely a condition is if a certain factor is present, compared to how likely it is if the factor is absent. For example, if someone is very obese, he or she has an odds ratio for diabetes of about 7, compared to someone of normal weight. If the odds ratio is 1, then the factor does not increase the risk at all. If the odds ratio is less than 1, the factor lowers the risk, and if the odds ratio is greater than 1, then the factor increases the risk.

The Danish scientists found that for people with definite polyneuropathy, the odds ratio linking this condition to statin use was 14.2; in other words, people on statins were fourteen times more likely to have polyneuropathy than people who had never been exposed to statins. For people who were treated with statins for two or more years, the odds ratio of definite polyneu-ropathy climbed to 26.4. The authors concluded that long-term statin use might substantially increase the risk of polyneuropathy. There have been many other reports from around the world of neuropathy related to statin use.

Do Statins Increase the Risk of Lou Gehrig's Disease?

Other postmarketing surveillance data (that is, infor-mation that has come to light after a drug has been released) have raised the disturbing possibility of in-creases in amyotrophic lateral sclerosis (ALS, or Lou Gehrig's disease) or ALS-like symptoms in people tak-ing statins. ALS is a disease of motor neurons, of un-known cause, that leads to muscle wasting, weakness, and eventual death. Fortunately, it is rare, affecting an estimated five in one hundred thousand individuals. There is no known cure. First reported in the journal *Drug Safety* in 2007,[18] the findings of a possible link be-tween an ALS-like syndrome and statins were based on data collected by the WHO Foundation Collaborating Centre for International Drug Monitoring. There were forty-three reports of ALS or ALS-like cases associated with statins described in this paper, and the authors conclude:

> The Individual Case Safety Reports presented in this investigation underline the possibility that severe, chronic, and persistent neuromuscular

problems may occur with a picture that may be difficult to distinguish from ALS and that it seems likely to be a class effect. We are concerned that the long-term and very broad use of these drugs is likely to lead to their being overlooked as a possible cause of neuromuscular events by both patients and health professionals.

Reported Side Effects from Statin Use

Muscle pain and muscle damage

Nerve damage (neuropathy)

Cognitive dysfunction

Tendonitis and tendon rupture

Joint pain and stiffness

Liver damage/liver function test abnormalities

Unmasking of mitochondrial dysfunction

Lou Gehrig's disease (amyotrophic lateral sclerosis)

Increase in diabetes

Congenital defects in children of women who took statins in pregnancy

---

Cancer and Statin Therapy

At least one randomized, controlled trial (RCT) of statins found an increased risk of cancer in the people treated with pravastatin, compared to placebo.[19] The subjects in this 2002 study, the Prospective Study of Pravastatin in the Elderly at Risk (PROSPER) trial, were all between the ages of seventy and eighty-two when they were recruited. They included 3,000 women and 2,804 men. The primary end point, a composite of nonfatal heart attack, death from coronary heart disease, and fatal and nonfatal stroke, was reduced 15 percent in those on pravastatin compared to placebo. That was a relative risk reduction; the absolute risk reduction was a paltry 2 percent. And, as was shown in other trials, men derived all the benefit; women had no reduction in their risk from treatment with the statin.

But over an average of 3.2 years of follow-up, the rate of new cancer diagnoses in the PROSPER study was 6.8 percent for those taking placebo and 8.5 percent for those taking pravastatin. If you were on pravastatin in this study, you had a 25 percent increased risk of developing cancer, which was statistically significant. Cancer death rates during the trial were 3.1 percent in the placebo group and 4 percent in the pravastatin group. This cancelled the mortality benefit of deaths due to coronary heart disease, which was 4.2 percent in the placebo group and 3.3 percent in the pravastatin group. There was no change in total mortality, implying that pravastatin treatment increased the risk of cancer death and decreased the risk of cardiac death. This increased risk of cancer was not found in other statin trials, where the average age of the participants was less than in PROSPER.

A more recent study published in 2010 in the journal *Cancer Prevention Research* found that statins did not lower the risk of colorectal cancer but appeared to increase the chances of developing precancerous colonic polyps.[20] (Most colon cancers develop from polyps, but not all polyps have the potential to become cancerous. However, the larger the polyp, the more likely it is to become cancerous.) Again, the risk seemed to correlate with the length of time the statins were taken: among those who took statins for three or more years, the risk of developing polyps was nearly 40 percent higher than for people not on statins. To be fair, this study was looking at whether or not the anti-inflammatory drug celecoxib (Celebrex) reduced the risk of colorectal polyps when compared to placebo. It was not directly assessing whether or not statin use, compared to placebo, had any effect on the risk of colorectal polyps, so the increased risk of colonic polyps in statin users was an unexpected finding.

Statins and the Risk of Diabetes

Finally, there is some indication that statin therapy may cause blood sugar to rise, thereby increasing the risk of diabetes. There was a significant increase in levels of hemoglobin A1c (a measure of average blood glucose levels over a three-month time span) in the Pravastatin or Atorvastatin Evaluation and Infection

Therapy (PROVE-IT) trial in the people randomized to high-dose atorvastatin (80 milligrams daily) compared to those assigned to moderate-dose pravastatin (40 milligrams daily).[21] All of the volunteers in this trial, before entering the study, had an acute coronary syndrome, defined as either an increase in anginal chest discomfort, or a heart attack.

In the JUPITER trial, the people who took 20 milligrams of rosuvastatin daily had a significant increase in hemoglobin A1c and a 25 percent greater risk of having a new diagnosis of diabetes compared to the people on placebo.[22] When British researchers looked at more than 90,000 participants in thirteen statin trials, they found that statins increased the risk of diabetes by 9 percent over an average of four years, and the risk was highest among older participants.[23] They calculated that treating 255 people with a statin for four years would cause one extra case of diabetes. And since about 40 million people in the United States take statins, an extra 156,000 people may develop diabetes as a result.

Statin Effects in a Large Population

In the spring of 2010, the *British Medical Journal* published an *observational study* of more than 2 million people in England and Wales who were treated with statins.[24] In observational studies, a group of people is observed over time, but no intervention is performed. For the *British Medical Journal* study, 368 general practitioners supplied data on statin use in their patients. A group of patients between the ages of thirty and eighty-four was identified from people registered in those practices between January 2002 and June 2008. Most received simvastatin (70.7 percent), with 22.3 percent receiving atorvastatin, 3.6 percent receiving pravastatin, 1.9 percent receiving rosuvastatin, and 1.4 percent receiving fluvastatin.

The study reported that statins did not increase the risk of Parkinson's disease, rheumatoid arthritis, dementia, blood clots in the veins, fractures from osteoporosis, melanoma (the deadliest form of skin cancer), and cancers of the stomach, kidney, lung, breast, and prostate. Although the risk of colon cancer was not increased (or lowered) in women who took statins, in men there was a lower risk of colon cancer in those treated with pravastatin but double the risk among men treated with rosuvastatin. Simvastatin was associated with a reduced risk of esophageal cancer in both men and women, but the effect was more apparent in men. The risk of esophageal cancer was also reduced in men who took atorvastatin. On the downside, statin use was associated with significantly increased risks of moderate or severe liver dysfunction, acute kidney failure, moderate or severe myopathy, and cataracts.

Statins and the Risk of Stroke

Statins have been shown to reduce the risk of strokes due to clots (thrombotic strokes) in some studies. But an often more devastating type of stroke, caused by bleeding into the brain, hemorrhagic stroke, is a different story. A study in the *Archives of Neurology* in 2011 showed that statins actually increase the risk of a second stroke in people who've had a hemorrhagic stroke.[25] The authors postulate that maybe having low cholesterol increases the risk of bleeding into the brain, or that the anticlotting effect of statins may increase the risk of brain hemorrhage. Once again, treatment with statins is shown to be a double-edged sword.

Statins in Pregnancy: Increased Risk of Congenital Defects

Before we leave the subject of statin side effects, a word about their use in pregnancy. Because cholesterol is vital to the normal development of the fetus, statins are said to be contraindicated in pregnancy. However, we are in the midst of an epidemic of diabetes, and more and more diabetic women are giving birth. Currently there are more than 12 million diabetic women in the United States. Diabetes is considered to be a coronary heart disease risk equivalent, (a CHD risk equivalent is a condition that puts you at very high risk for having a cardiac event) and current guidelines suggest that diabetics be treated to reduce their LDL cholesterol below 100, which almost always requires a medicine, most often a statin. Therefore, diabetic women, many of childbearing age, are often put on these drugs.

A study published in 2004 looked at congenital defects among the babies of 214 women who had taken statins during pregnancy.[26] The authors reported that exposure to statins was associated with five cases of fetal death, four cases of low birth weight, and twenty-two cases of congenital defects. These defects included severe defects of the central nervous system like spina bifida, abnormalities of the arms and legs, cleft lip or palate, and severe abnormalities of the gastrointestinal and genitourinary tracts.

Statin Use in Children

While we are on the subject of children: despite the chilling evidence that long-term use of statins can cause serious harm, Big Pharma is pushing to have more and more children put on statins. Due to the epidemic of obesity affecting children (as well as adults), more and more youngsters are being diagnosed with diabetes, abnormal levels of blood fats, and high blood pressure. As reported in New-Medical.net in 2010, Pfizer announced that the European Commission had approved a chewable form of Lipitor for children over the age of ten.[27] (The European Commission, head-quartered in Brussels, is one of the main institutions of the European Union. It is responsible for drafting proposals for new laws and represents the interests of the union as a whole.) I find it unconscionable to treat children with a drug that has serious side effects, when diet and exercise can achieve the same benefits with no risk at all. But apparently not all physicians share my concern.

Downplaying the Harm, Hyping the Benefits of Statins

So, despite the well-publicized benefits of statins, they are not without risk of serious side effects. As with every other decision about drugs, you and your doctor must weigh the potential advantages against the potential harm. Unfortunately, the authors of statin studies and their sponsors in Big Pharma tend to hype the benefits and downplay the harm. The studies last for only a few years, so adverse effects that occur after long-term statin use may not be apparent during the short time span of most clinical trials.

Further muddying the waters is the huge amount of money at stake. Billions of dollars of Big Pharma profit are on the line. Is it any wonder that the truth is often obscured? And can we be confident that researchers on Big Pharma's payroll are reporting the results of these trials accurately? What exactly is the relationship between Big Pharma and the medical establishment today? Do we have reason to be concerned? These questions will be explored later in this book.

Chapter 4

Why Can't a Woman Be More Like a Man? Gender Differences and Statin Use

B.P. was a successful television writer who was put on a statin when she was fifty-two years old. Her total cholesterol was 201, and she had high blood pressure, but she didn't smoke, was not diabetic, did not have a family history of premature coronary heart disease, and had never exhibited any symptoms of heart disease. Within six months, she was experiencing severe pain in her legs, fatigue, ringing in her ears, confusion, and memory loss. She also developed jaundice, shoulder pain, frequent falls, and lost all interest in sex.

After an airplane flight, she developed urine "the color of Coca-Cola." B.P. went to a hospital, where her CPK muscle enzyme level was found to be elevated. But she was not told to stop the statin medicine, and after about fourteen months on simvastatin (Zocor), she was unable to work. One time she caused a fire in her home by forgetting that the stove was on. She found it impossible to sew, which she had formerly enjoyed. Worried that she was developing Alzheimer's, B.P. went to a clinic that specialized in this disease. Testing revealed that her cognitive skills were at 69 percent of normal. She was also diagnosed with neuropathy in her hands and feet. She had such severe sciatic pain that she could sit for only fifteen minutes at a time. Finally, her husband, who is a scientist, said to her, "You are being poisoned." She stopped the simvastatin that she had been taking for twenty-eight months, and her neuropathy resolved, but her memory loss and muscle pain persist. She subsequently had a muscle biopsy that demonstrated mitochondrial myopathy.

B.P. says of the statin she took: "It's destroyed me. I've lost my income; I've lost everything. I've lost my friends because I don't remember them." She tells me, "You need to quote Hitler: the bigger the lie, the more people believe it."

———

F.E. is a delightful woman who first came to see me in 1985. She'd suffered what was described as a "small heart attack" and was continuing to have chest discomfort that sounded like angina. I performed a heart catheterization, which revealed a complete blockage in one coronary artery, but her other coronary artery did not have any significant buildup of plaque. She was continued on medicine to treat her angina.

Nine years later, in 1996, she noted an increase in the number of angina attacks she was having. I performed another cardiac catheterization, which showed a nearly 50 percent narrowing in two other branches of the coronary arteries. At that point, I started her on pravastatin (Pravachol) in an attempt to lower her cholesterol. F.E.'s

LDL cholesterol was 140, and with treatment it dropped to 86. She took the statin for eleven months and then developed constipation, headaches, and abdominal pain, which resolved when she stopped the pravastatin. She was unwilling to go back on this medicine but was willing to take a low dose of another statin, atorvastatin (Lipitor). However, her abdominal pain recurred, so after just a few months, she discontinued the atorvastatin. F.E. agreed to try pravastatin again but soon developed diffuse muscle pain. She stopped pravastatin in May 1998 and has not taken a statin since then.

Ten years later, in October 2008, she again noted an increase in her angina and underwent another cardiac catheterization. She had more significant blockages and had four stents placed in her coronary arteries. F.E. continues to have mild, stable angina, but she has not had another heart attack, and at age ninety-two, she still lives independently.

D.D. came to my office for the first time in 2002, when she was ninety-two, complaining of heart palpitations. She was taking a baby aspirin each day and a diuretic, or "water pill," every other day for swelling of her ankles. Although her parents had died in their sixties, she had four siblings who were also in their nineties. D.D. had never smoked, did not have high blood pressure, and was not diabetic.

Her palpitations were found to be due to benign extra beats and she continued living independently. In 2004 she was found to have an underactive thyroid gland

and was started on thyroid hormone. Two years later, her primary care doctor obtained a cholesterol panel. Her total cholesterol was 266, her triglycerides were 169, her HDL cholesterol was 66, and her LDL cholesterol was 165. He gave D.D. a prescription for a statin medicine, but she was unwilling to take it. She saw me in the office a few months later, and I reassured her that she did not need to be on a statin. She is now 102 years old and has no signs or symptoms of heart disease.

In the Oscar-winning movie *My Fair Lady*, Professor Henry Higgins, in a fit of pique at the apparent ingratitude of his student Eliza Doolittle, erupts into a witty, albeit misogynistic song, inquiring of his sidekick Colonel Hugh Pickering, "Why can't a woman be more like a man? / Men are so honest, so thoroughly square; / eternally noble, historically fair."

Medical science took Professor Higgins's attitude, an apt summary of the early-twentieth-century's stance toward women, a step further, deciding that for all intents and purposes women *were* just like men—with the exception noted below. The scientific community felt that you could use men as subjects in clinical trials and apply the results willy-nilly to women. When I was in medical school, my professors took the "bikini approach" to women's health: women's health meant breasts and reproductive organs. Otherwise the prototypical patient was presented as a man, and the term *gender medicine* had not been coined yet .

The last few decades have seen a flowering of

interest in the gender-specific aspects of a whole slew of diseases. Much remains to be learned, and more needs to be done to ensure that women are included in meaningful numbers in the clinical trials that tell us how to prevent and treat diseases. Because as we shall see, women often react differently to medicines, have more side effects, and derive less benefit than men do. Statins are a classic example of this.

It wasn't until 1986 that the National Institutes of Health (NIH) encouraged the inclusion of women in clinical trials. Seven years later, when nothing much had changed, Congress passed a law mandating that women be recruited for medical research: the National Institutes of Health Revitalization Act of 1993, Public Law 103–43. But even so, the percentage of women in most clinical trials of heart disease has been woefully low. And as stated in a report from the prestigious Institute of Medicine, a nonprofit organization that provides information on improving health:

> The entire issue of inclusion of women in clinical trials would be moot if men and women responded identically to therapy. Current knowledge about differential response is incomplete. However, exclusion of women from clinical research that establishes the safety, efficacy, and mode of administration of drugs or other interventions prevents physicians from having sufficient information to make informed judgments about treatment of women.[1]

Primary Prevention with Statins in Women

So let's take a closer look at statin studies, and let's start with primary prevention trials, those that recruit healthy people and try to prevent a first cardiovascular event. The first primary prevention trial of statins and atherosclerotic cardiovascular disease did not include any women at all. Reported in 1995, the so-called WOSCOPS trial, from the West of Scotland Coronary Prevention Study Group, randomized 6,595 men with no history of heart attack but high levels of cholesterol to either pravastatin or placebo. The primary end points were a nonfatal heart attack or death from coronary heart disease (CHD). There was a relative risk reduction of 31 percent in the men treated with statins compared to placebo. But if you look at the absolute risk reduction, it was a mere 2.2 percent.[2]

The next primary prevention trial to be reported, and the first that included women, was the Air Force/ Texas Coronary Atherosclerosis Prevention Study (AFCAPS/TexCAPS),[3] which randomized 5,608 men, ages forty-five to seventy-three, and 997 women, ages fifty-five to seventy-three, with average levels of total and LDL cholesterol but low levels of HDL cholesterol (the good kind) to either lovastatin (Mevacor) or placebo. The higher minimum age for women was chosen because we know that women tend to develop signs of ASCVD about ten years later than men do.

The primary end points in this study were not as hard as they were in WOSCOPS, because, in addition to nonfatal heart attack and CHD death, they included unstable angina—a diagnosis that is subject to more inaccuracy than death or heart attack. Among the almost one thousand women in this trial, there were seven end points in the lovastatin-treated group and thirteen end points in the placebo-treated group, but given the very small numbers of end points, this difference was not statistically significant. (If you look only at the hard end points of cardiac death or heart attack, there were no cardiac deaths among the women on placebo and one cardiac death among those on lovastatin. There were six nonfatal heart attacks among the women taking placebo and four nonfatal heart attacks among those on lovastatin.) In contrast, there were 109 end points among men on lovastatin compared to 170 end points in men on placebo—and this difference was statistically significant. Despite these results, I have attended talks where the lecturer reports that statin therapy in women in the AFCAPS/TexCAPS trial lowered risk by about 50 percent! Overall, the relative risk reduction for the whole study population was 37 percent, but the absolute risk reduction was 2 percent. As you'll notice, these results were very similar to the WOSCOPS results.

The next primary prevention trial of statins was the Anglo-Scandinavian Cardiac Outcomes Trial-Lipid Lowering Arm (ASCOT-LLA).[4] The ASCOT trial was designed to see if a newer blood pressure medicine called amlodipine (Norvasc) was superior to an older blood pressure medicine, the beta-blocker atenolol (Tenormin). A subset of people enrolled in the ASCOT trial, who did not have very high cholesterol levels, were then chosen for a substudy in which they were treated with either atorvastatin or placebo. This sub-study was given the acronym ASCOT-LLA. The men and women in this trial had to have high blood pressure and at least three other risk factors for CHD. In other words, even though they didn't have documented heart disease, they were at high risk. The study enrolled 1,942 women and 8,363 men ranging in age from forty to seventy-nine years. The participants were followed for the occurrence of the primary end point: either nonfatal heart attack or death due to CHD. Overall, the relative risk reduction in people on statins compared to placebo was 36 percent, but the absolute risk reduction was 2.1 percent.

At the end of the trial, there had been 100 primary end point events in the atorvastatin group compared to 154 end point events in the placebo group. This difference was statistically significant. But the benefit occurred exclusively in men. There were 19 end point events in women on atorvastatin and 17 end point events in women on placebo. Clearly, the women who took atorvastatin in this study saw *no* reduction in their risk of a cardiac event.

But you would never know this from Pfizer's television and print advertisements for Caduet, the brand name of the combination drug containing atorvastatin and the high blood pressure medicine amlodipine. The advertisements showed a healthy-looking woman who appeared no older than forty extolling the benefits of Caduet. And yet the ASCOT-LLA trial that studied these same two drugs failed to show that women derived *any* benefit whatsoever. The same complaint was made against commercials for Pfizer's drug Lipitor, and they were eventually pulled from television. Perhaps this had something to do with a class action suit that accused the pharmaceutical company of devising "a promotional scheme to boost sales of its anticholesterol drug Lipitor by misleading women and seniors about the link between the drug and heart disease."[5]

Pfizer also got into trouble for its Lipitor advertisements that featured Dr. Robert Jarvik, the inventor of the Jarvik-7 artificial heart. Speaking as if he were a physician who prescribes Lipitor (he's never been a practicing physician), Jarvik touted the benefits of taking Lipitor. The commercials were yanked from television when a congressional probe started looking into whether they were misleading.

If you add up the number of end points in women in these two trials, AFCAPS/TexCAPS and ASCOT-LLA, you come up with these numbers: there were twenty-six end points in women on statins and thirty end points in women on placebo. The number of women in the two trials totaled 2,939, and they were equally divided between statin and placebo groups. You don't have to be a statistician to realize that the difference between these two treatments is not statistically significant. Despite this, many physicians, who hadn't read the entire articles reporting these studies, started prescribing statins to healthy women with elevated levels of LDL cholesterol. Why? Because they thought the results in men also applied to women. This is not a scientifically valid conclusion. Thousands of women were treated with statins when they didn't need to be.

The JUPITER Trial Results in Women

Now we come to the JUPITER trial, which was touted as the first primary prevention trial that showed a benefit for statin therapy in healthy women. When the study was proposed, statins were in wide use in people who had atherosclerotic cardiovascular disease, or who were at very high risk because of diabetes or multiple risk factors. However, there was still a great deal of skepticism about the use of statins for primary prevention, despite the "positive" results of the three earlier primary prevention trials: WOSCOPS, AFCAPS/Tex-CAPS, and ASCOT-LLA. In particular, the effectiveness of primary prevention with statins in women had not been proven.

The stakes for Big Pharma were high: if statins could be proven to prevent cardiovascular events in healthy people, then the numbers of men and women whose physicians would advise to them to go on statins would take a quantum leap. In fact, as I've already noted, when the results of JUPITER were used to justify the FDA's decision in 2010 to expand the indications for taking rosuvastatin (Crestor), it was estimated that six and a half million healthy people would be added to the rolls of those taking statins. And since Crestor costs about $3.50 per pill, we're talking about $1,277.50 per person, per year—or a whopping $8.3 billion a year. When you add the cost of monitoring for adverse effects, the total jumps to over $9 billion annually, and that's even before you add in the cost of the hsCRP blood test, which can vary from about $20 to $80. According to Dr. James Stein, director of preventive cardiology at the University of Wisconsin School of Medicine and Public Health, that comes to a cost of about $557,000 per life saved.[6]

The JUPITER trial was performed at 1,315 sites in twenty-six countries. To be included in the study, participants had to be free of diagnosed cardiovascular disease, could not be diabetic, and had to have an LDL cholesterol of less than 130 plus evidence of increased inflammation as measured by the hsCRP blood test. The trial was funded by AstraZeneca, the makers of rosuvastatin.

The investigators did a very good job of including women, who made up 38 percent of the 17,802 participants. The men in the trial had to be at least fifty years old, and the women had to be at least sixty. This is the kind of detail that practicing physicians often overlook or are unaware of. They hear that a trial had a positive result and begin to put even healthy people in their thirties on statins if their cholesterol is one or two points higher than "goal." I see this in my office every week, and it makes me want to tear my hair out.

To much fanfare in the press, it was announced at the American Heart Association's annual scientific meeting in 2008 that the JUPITER trial had been discontinued prematurely after a median follow-up of only 1.9 years (the trial had been scheduled to last up to five years) for "benefit" in reducing the primary end point among the statin-treated group.

The primary end point in the JUPITER trial was a composite of (1) heart attack, (2) stroke, (3) a revascularization procedure such as bypass surgery or angioplasty/stent, (4) hospitalization for unstable angina, or (5) death from heart disease. The authors reported that the rates of the primary end point were 0.77 per one hundred person years of follow-up in the statin group and 1.36 per one hundred person years in the placebo group. A person-year of follow-up means that you have followed one person for one year. Therefore, one hundred person years of follow-up means that you followed one hundred people for one year, or, were it not extremely impractical and unlikely, one person for one hundred years.

By the end of the study, 75 percent of the participants were still taking their study drug, but the analysis was by intention to treat—that is, you were counted in whichever group you were originally assigned to even if you had stopped taking your study drug. The authors noted that when the study was stopped prematurely, 142 first major cardiovascular events had occurred in the rosuvastatin group, as compared with 251 in the placebo group. The investigators reported that the benefit of rosuvastatin was consistent among all the subgroups, including women and minorities.

I was very intrigued by these results when they were published in the *New England Journal of Medicine* in November 2008.[7] This was the very first time that a trial was said to show that statin use in healthy women lowered their risk of having a cardiac event. But the study just gave the absolute numbers of events in the *whole group*, not in the subgroups. And even though the authors said that the relative risk reduction in women (46 percent) was similar to that in men (42 percent), I was curious to learn what the *absolute* numbers of primary end points were in the two groups of women. So, perhaps naively, I emailed principal investigator Dr. Paul Ridker, explaining that I lectured frequently on women and heart disease, and asked for the numbers of primary end points in women so that I could update my slides. I received an email from his secretary promising me that they would send me those numbers shortly, but despite my repeated requests, they never arrived.

Finally, in February 2010 a separate article appeared in the journal *Circulation*, detailing the results of the JUPITER trial in women.[8]

You will recall that in the overall group, the event rates of the primary end point were 0.77 and 1.36 per one hundred person years, comparing rosuvastatin to placebo. Broken down by sex, the comparable numbers were 0.88 and 1.54 for men, and 0.57 and 1.04 for women.

In other words, women had much lower event rates than men, even though they were older. The median age for women in JUPITER was sixty-eight versus sixty-three for men, but no woman was under sixty at entry into the study. In addition, women were less likely than men to be white, were heavier, and more of them had high blood pressure. They were also more likely to have the metabolic syndrome. (It bears repeating that the metabolic syndrome is diagnosed if you have three out of five of the following: abdominal obesity (a waist measurement of more than thirty-five inches in a woman or forty inches in a man); a fasting blood sugar of 100 milligrams per deciliter of blood (110 mg/dl) or more; a fasting triglycerides level of 150 milligrams per deciliter or more; a blood pressure of 130/85 or higher; and an HDL cholesterol of under 50 in a woman or under 40 in a man.)

This constellation of risk factors is actually much more common in people with atherosclerosis than high levels of LDL cholesterol are. But perhaps because you can "cure" the metabolic syndrome with physical exercise and a heart-healthy diet, it receives very little attention from Big Pharma. The drug companies would prefer us to focus on LDL cholesterol because they have statin drugs that are quite effective in lowering that risk factor. But I digress.

Women also had higher levels of hsCRP (4.6 versus 4.1 in men), and women had slightly but statistically significant higher levels of LDL cholesterol (109 for women and 108 for men). As would be expected, women also had higher levels of HDL cholesterol, by about 10. (Remember that normal levels of HDL cholesterol are 50 and above for women and 40 and above for men.) Small but statistically significant differences were also noted in fasting blood sugar (lower in women), although hemoglobin A1c, a measure of average blood sugar over three months, was lower in men. The one risk factor that was significantly more common in men than women in JUPITER was smoking. Only 7.6 percent of women were current smokers, while 21 percent of men were.

So despite being older and having generally higher levels of various risk factors, women had lower event rates than men whether they were in the statin-treated group or the placebo group.

Now let's take a look at some absolute numbers. You may recall that there were 251 primary end points in the placebo group and 142 events in the rosuvastatin group. Broken down by sex, there were 181 primary end points in men on placebo versus 103 primary end points in men on rosuvastatin. As we noted above, this translates to event rates per one hundred person years in men of 1.54 versus 0.88, placebo versus statin. There were 70 primary end points in women on placebo and 39 events in women on rosuvastatin. This translates to event rates per one hundred person years in women of 1.04 versus 0.57, placebo versus statin. Whether on active drug or placebo, women had strikingly lower event rates than men.

Where it gets *really* interesting is if we break the composite primary end point into its individual components. In women, unlike men, there were no statistically significant reductions in the risk of fatal or nonfatal heart attacks, or fatal or nonfatal strokes. (Neither men nor women in the JUPITER trial had a reduction in their mortality rate from taking the statin.) The only part of the composite primary end point that showed a significant benefit for rosuvastatin in women was in the need for revascularization or unstable angina. But these are softer end points than stroke, heart attack, and death, which have strict criteria before they can be diagnosed. As I said previously, we doctors don't often get death wrong. But whether or not to refer someone for a revascularization procedure, be it a balloon angioplasty/stent or a coronary bypass operation, is a decision for which different doctors have different thresholds. And I'm inclined to believe, although I don't know it for a fact, that these procedures are performed more frequently in the United States and the United Kingdom than in Bulgaria, although people from all three of these countries participated in the JUPITER trial. In fact, it's fair to say that revascularization and hospitalization are not really end points. They are decisions made by physicians. It may be that they were added to the composite primary end point in order to have a sufficient number of events to achieve statistical significance.

Just to give you one example from my own practice, I have a patient we'll call Millie who is in her eighties. She complained of chest pain that lasted for hours, was not brought on or exacerbated by exertion or emotional upset, was not relieved by nitroglycerin, and was not associated with characteristic changes in her electrocardiogram. I was quite confident that Millie's pain was not angina and suggested she discuss with her primary care doctor having a workup for other causes, such as acid reflux disease,.

One night her pain became so severe, that she called 911 and an ambulance took her to a hospital where I am not on staff. There she was seen by another cardiologist who did a heart catheterization. This revealed a narrowing in one of the branches of her left coronary artery, which was promptly dilated with a balloon and a stent. The procedure did nothing to relieve her pain, which did not go away until she was treated for acid reflux disease. But if Millie had been in the JUPITER trial, she would have been diagnosed as someone with unstable angina and an arterial revascularization.

We know that statins can cause the smooth muscle of arteries to relax. And this, similar to the action of the medicine nitroglycerin, may explain why, compared to placebo, people taking rosuvastatin in the JUPITER trial had less unstable angina than people taking placebo. It's certainly plausible that this accounts for the beneficial effect, but the fact that this was the only "significant" benefit in women on rosuvastatin compared to placebo lessens the validity of the study, in my opinion, and makes me unwilling to extend statin therapy to large numbers of healthy women.

Given all of these differences between the outcomes in women and men, the number needed to treat for five years to prevent one primary end point calculates to be thirty-six women (compared to twenty-two men). So thirty-five of those women treated for five years would derive *no* measurable benefit, at a cost of $223,562.50 (assuming a cost per pill of $3.50). Is that how we want to spend our limited health care dollars?

The occurrence of serious adverse events was said to be similar in men and women in both the placebo and statin-treated groups. Serious adverse events, including muscle weakness, stiffness, pain, myopathy, newly diagnosed cancer, death from cancer, and kidney, gastrointestinal, or bleeding disorder, were similar in men and women across treatments. Men did have a statistically significant increase in the risk of liver function abnormalities in the group treated with rosuvastatin compared to placebo, which was not seen in women. With respect to the development of diabetes, a higher incidence was observed in women treated with rosuvastatin compared to placebo (1.53 versus 1.03 per one hundred person years, respectively), compared to men (1.36 versus 1.20 per one hundred person years). Since diabetes increases cardiovascular disease risk in women more than in men, this is a disturbing statistic, one that has not received nearly enough attention from the medical profession or the media.

Finally, an analysis of participants under age sixty-five compared to those sixty-five or older showed no statistically significant benefit in lowering the risk of a primary end point in women in the under-sixty-five age group, which numbered 1,942 women. This difference based on age was not seen in men. Despite this, in expanding the indications for rosuvastatin, the FDA approved its use in women beginning at age sixty if they have an hsCRP of 2 or more, and one other risk factor for ASCVD.

Controversy over the FDA Decision

The decision to expand the indications for rosuvastatin has been controversial. Dr. Mark Hlatky, a professor at Stanford University School of Medicine, opined in an article in the March 30, 2010, *New York Times,* "It's a good thing to be skeptical about whether there may be long-term harm from healthy people taking a drug like this." And Dr. Rita Redberg of the University of California had this to say in *Time* magazine on March 29, 2010: "There are millions of women on a drug with no known benefit and risks that are detrimental to their lifestyle—and no one is talking about it. Why?"

Why indeed? Could it have anything to do with the billions of dollars in play? As noted by Dr. Marcia Angell, former editor of the *New England Journal of Medicine,* in her book *The Truth About the Drug Companies: How They Deceive Us and What to Do About It,* the combined profits of the ten largest drug companies in the Fortune 500 in 2002 amounted to $35.9 billion, which was more than the combined profits of the remaining 490 companies ($33.7 billion).

Perhaps the best reason to take the results of the JUPITER study with a grain of salt is apparent at the very end of the report—where the authors disclose their financial stakes. Dr. Paul Ridker, the lead author, receives grant support and consulting and/or lecture fees from the makers of rosuvastatin, AstraZeneca, and nine other large pharmaceutical companies. He also holds the patent on the high-sensitivity CRP test. Of the other ten medical doctors who were coauthors, only one did not report any income from grants, consulting fees, or lecture fees from Big Pharma. The paper states, "No other potential conflict of interest relevant to this article was reported." *No other?* Are those admitted not sufficient? But the story doesn't end there.

A few months after the publication of the gender-specific results of the JUPITER trial, an article criticizing the trial was published in the journal *Archives of Internal Medicine*.[9] The lead author, Michel de Lorgeril, was a principal investigator of the Lyon Diet Heart Study, which will be discussed in the next chapter. The authors pointed out several methodological problems with JUPITER, including the lack of information on which specific end points were used to justify the early termination of the study. Remember, the trial was stopped for "benefit" after a median follow-up of only 1.9 years. It was recently shown that truncated trials appear to show greater benefits than trials that are not stopped early. In fact, the original article contains a graph showing all-cause mortality. The lines that represented deaths in the treated subjects versus the control subjects diverged initially but appeared to be converging when the trial was ended. This suggests that the borderline significant difference between the groups might have disappeared if follow-up had been longer. And as de Lorgeril and his colleagues noted: "Strangely, in a subsequent article that was apparently written to defuse the controversy, the all-cause mortality curves were truncated so that the previous converging portion was no longer displayed."

The de Lorgeril article also pointed out that although an unequivocal reduction in cardiovascular mortality was announced when the trial was ended prematurely in March 2008, the "absence of cardiovascular mortality data in the published article is striking." The original article that gave the JUPITER results never presented the number of deaths from cardiovascular causes. But de Lorgeril and his colleagues teased it out from the data on fatal and nonfatal heart attacks and strokes, which were given. And lo and behold, that number came to twelve in the treated group and twelve in the placebo group. Clearly, there was no difference, and as the article observed, "such a lack of effect on cardiovascular mortality associated with a strong effect on nonfatal complications strongly suggests a bias in the data set and should have led to the continuation of the trial rather than to its premature ending."

Another anomaly in the JUPITER study was that the ratio of fatal heart attack to nonfatal heart attack was described by the authors of the *Archives of Internal Medicine* article as "incredibly low," especially in the placebo group. From various studies, we know that out of one hundred people who have heart attacks, an average of fifty die almost immediately or within the next several weeks. In the JUPITER trial, the case fatality rate (the rate of deaths within a group, over a defined period of time) was 8.8 percent in the placebo group and 29 percent in the rosuvastatin group. Again, this clinical inconsistency suggests a major flaw in the study.

An earlier critic of the study, Dr. Paul S. Chan of the Saint Luke's Mid America Heart and Vascular Institute, using data from the original paper, calculated that there were thirty-one cardiovascular deaths in the rosuvastatin group, and thirty-seven in the placebo group, not a significant difference.[10] Because twelve deaths in each group were due to fatal heart attack or fatal stroke, it is unclear what caused these other deaths. Ridker, responding to this question, said that they resulted from "vascular causes such as aneurysm rupture." It is not credible that there were more fatal aneurysm ruptures than heart attacks in either group. And even more surprising is the lack of any data on *sudden cardiac death (SCD—death occurring within a short period of time, usually one hour, of the onset of an illness or symptoms)* in the JUPITER trial. In fact, SCD is never mentioned, even though it usually accounts for 65 percent to 70 percent of all cardiac deaths.

Cardiovascular mortality in JUPITER appears to be very low compared to the total mortality that was observed: between 5 percent and 18 percent, depending on how it was calculated, whereas one would expect that cardiovascular mortality would be about 40 percent of total mortality. The data in JUPITER are therefore not epidemiologically consistent, and this may have been due at least partially to the early termination of the trial.

De Lorgeril and his colleagues also point out that most of the authors of the original JUPITER article had financial ties to AstraZeneca, the sponsor, and that the sponsor played a "pervasive" role in the study: "The sponsor collected the trial data and monitored the study sites." This is clearly stated in the paper. Yet when I spoke to several AstraZeneca representatives in my quest for the data on women in the study, they denied that they had access to the data. As noted by De Lorgeril and his colleagues, "The results of the JUPITER trial support concerns that commercially sponsored clinical trials are at risk of poor quality and bias."

So the answer to the question "Do you believe in JUPITER?" is no—I certainly don't. It is a deeply flawed trial, and the FDA was grossly in error when it expanded the indications for using rosuvastatin to an estimated six and a half million healthy Americans.

Why Are Statins Less Effective in Women?

I hope I have convinced you that women derive less benefit from statin drugs than men do. But why is that? A study published in 2001 may hold at least part of the answer to that question.[11] This clinical trial recruited more than 2,400 healthy men and more than 2,000 healthy women between the ages of forty and sixty-four and followed them for an average of nineteen years. Everyone had measurements of their total cholesterol, LDL cholesterol, HDL cholesterol, and *non-HDL cholesterol* (if this number is elevated, it means that triglycerides are elevated). The end point of this study was death due to cardiovascular disease (CVD), a very hard end point. In men, high total cholesterol, high non-HDL cholesterol, high LDL cholesterol, and low HDL cholesterol were all significantly associated with an increased risk of CVD death. But in women, only low HDL cholesterol and high non-HDL cholesterol were significantly associated with an increased risk of CVD death. In women, even levels of LDL cholesterol more than 190 were associated with only a small, statistically nonsignificant increased risk of dying of cardiovascular disease.

So the fact that women derive less benefit from a

medicine that mainly lowers LDL cholesterol may be due to the fact that elevated LDL cholesterol is less harmful to women than it is to men.

Even in secondary prevention trials, the evidence that women benefit from statin therapy is not nearly as convincing as the evidence that men do. The numbers of people who have participated in secondary prevention trials of statins is in the tens of thousands. Some of the research studies have shown a statistically significant benefit in women, but others have not.

If you total up the event rates in five large secondary prevention trials in which statins were compared to placebo (involving 32,956 men and 11,001 women), the event rates decreased from 25.5 percent in men on placebo to 19.5 percent in men on statins. In women, the comparable event rates were 17 percent in women on placebo and 13.9 percent in women on statins. The results in both men and women were statistically significant, but both the absolute risk reduction and the relative risk reduction were lower in women. In fact, the 17 percent event rate seen in women taking placebo was lower than the 19.5 percent event rate seen in men taking statins.

———

So, to sum up: statins reduce the risk of recurrent cardiac events in women who have established vascular disease, but the drugs are less effective in this regard for women than they are for men. In women under the age of sixty-five who don't have established vascular disease, we have *zero* evidence that statin treatment lowers

their risk of having a cardiac event. This holds true
even if we factor in the results of the JUPITER trial.
And women experience more side effects from statins
than men do.

That's why extending the use of statins to millions
of healthy women, with normal cholesterol levels but
evidence of inflammation, based on one short-term
study (JUPITER) makes no sense at all—unless you are
a Big Pharma company standing to make millions of
dollars in profits from the sale of these drugs.

What really gets my dander up is that you can lower
your risk of heart disease without taking any drugs at
all and, therefore, without encountering *any* side effects. How to go about doing just that is the subject of
the next chapter.

Chapter 5

So What Am I to Do?
Practical Lifestyle Approaches
to Heart Health

One of my patients penned this story of his experiences with statins. He remains healthy, vigorous, and off statins to this day, on the diet discussed in this chapter.

————

I am a fifty-eight-year-old man who is slim, physically active, healthy. As is the case with two of my three siblings, the cholesterol in my blood—particularly the one of the not so desirable kind—is moderately elevated. My GP started me on a statin in 2001; atorvastatin (Lipitor) at 10 milligrams per day worked to his complete satisfaction and to mine.

Or so I thought. In 2005 I started experiencing paresthesia and joint pain, mostly in the legs and arms. These symptoms, albeit mild, were unusual, and I consulted with my GP and with a neurologist. Neither of them thought much of it. Statin was not on anybody's mind; I had been taking it for four years, and my liver enzymes, checked twice yearly, were fine.

In the spring of 2009, my health took a turn for the

worse. I became incapacitated, in more than one way. When getting out of bed every morning, the pain in my ankles made putting my feet on the ground an unpleasant experience. Walking up the stairs would be so uncomfortable that I got into the habit of climbing on all fours. This required a bit of maneuvering on my part, lest my wife witness the strange performance. The joint pain, now accompanied by muscle ache, was such that I had to discontinue my regular exercising on the NordicTrack, as well as all other forms of exercise and sport.

At about the same time, some cognitive disorders set in. As a university professor, I am held to high standards in my teaching and research. In the past, my brain had always lived up to the job. Now my mental faculties were beginning to show unusual—and quite unpleasant—signs of weakness. Every new scientific project seemed to peter out in my hands. My productivity as a researcher, which, over a period of several years had gradually slowed down, now ground to a halt. That was hard enough. But I also was deeply concerned about my PhD students, who depended on my guidance for their own research—and careers. By the end of the spring semester of 2009, the short-term-memory impairment was such that even teaching an easy course was fraught with difficulty.

Along with cognitive dysfunction came depression. Surely, doing so poorly at work was cause enough for some depression. Yet I sank into a depression so deep that I now think it must have been caused, at least in part, by a disruption of some of the brain mechanisms that normally control emotions. I became chronically *and inexplicably angry, and started avoiding people, whether friends or colleagues. Strangely, I was interpreting the changes in my body and brain as a form of accelerated aging process. I was witnessing my own gradual loss of interest in life: research was gone; teaching was difficult, even painful; my marriage was suffering direly; exercising was out of the question—even gardening had become too much of an effort; listening to music or playing the piano had lost its taste, and so had going to a museum or an exhibit. I felt, almost physically, that the multiple threads that had connected me to the world throughout my life were now being severed one after another, at an oddly accelerated pace. I became obsessed with death and began to contemplate the possibility that I wouldn't make it to the age of sixty.*

Among other things, I had lost the faculty for making a sound judgment and/or the ability to make a decision and act on it. Indeed I did not, in that entire period of time, seek medical or psychological help, as I would normally do for any serious discomfort or health concern, be it physical or emotional.

Fast-forward to July 21 of that year: my wake-up call rings at five in the morning. I am in a hotel room in Kloten, a small town near Zurich Airport, and have to catch an early plane to fly back home. I grew up in France, and hiking in the Alps is, hands down, my favorite way of storing up energy in the summer. This time, too, I feel better after two weeks in Davos. Yet I am not well. I must face it: if even Switzerland can't work its magic, something must be seriously amiss. But what? What?

Possibly because my brain was somehow jarred by the early wake-up call, possibly an effect of Switzerland's magic after all, the memory of an old dinner conversation comes back to me. The wife of a colleague is telling me, "I hear you started taking statins. You should watch out; they will do bad things to your muscles." I had shrugged it off. How strange that this seven-year-old conversation is popping up now out of nowhere. Well, I have fifteen minutes before going down to breakfast, and the room has wireless Internet access. I boot up my laptop and type in "statin and muscle aches."

That morning, I missed the airport shuttle. I took a cab. Twenty Swiss francs well spent: I knew I would never touch a statin again in my life.

Within days, I felt markedly better. Within a few weeks, both the joint pain and the muscle aches had cleared. The paresthesia, which had been the first symptom to appear, lingered a bit longer. The lifting of the depression was nothing short of spectacular. In short order, I started attending seminars again, I resumed my scientific research, I started giving talks. In the eighteen months after July 2009, I wrote four papers, three of which are now published. I got my PhD students back on track; one of them defended his thesis in the spring of 2010 and landed a position at a good university.

The very last symptom to go was a reflex: that of reaching for the railing every time I went up or down the stairs, any stairs—as short and easy as the four steps to my back porch. I became aware of that deeply ingrained gesture only a few months after going off the statin, when I found myself, day after day, stopping my hand in *midcourse, as grabbing the railing had become unnecessary.*

My Rollerblades and my snowboard, which had been gathering dust in the basement and which I thought I might never use again, are back in service. I have every intention of continuing to use them into old age, just as I have every intention of keeping my blood cholesterol just as it is now: moderately higher than it "should" be. Into old age.

Diets and Why Fats Were Demonized (Unfairly)

Ancel Keys was an American scientist who lived for almost 101 years. It's a safe bet that he knew a thing or two about healthy eating. Dr. Keys was the first to popularize what has come to be known as the Mediterranean diet. He and his colleagues studied the diets of more than twelve thousand men residing in countries around the world; they also obtained data on death rates and causes of death. The Seven Countries Study, begun in the 1950s, showed that people who lived on the Greek island of Crete had the world's lowest rate of death from cardiac disease and the longest life expectancy, despite a diet that was high in fat. The hook was that just about the only fat in the Cretan diet was olive oil. Now, the people of Crete didn't think they were on any special diet. The foods they ate were the foods their ancestors had eaten for generations. They consumed vegetables, fruits, whole grains, beans, goat cheese, nuts, olive oil, bread, seafood, red wine with meals, and very little meat. It's another safe bet that, at least in the 1950s and 1960s, they weren't subsisting on Whoppers, Kentucky Fried Chicken, potato chips, cotton candy, and milk shakes. Nowadays we call the diet Cretans consumed in the 1950s the Mediterranean diet.

Key Components of the Mediterranean Diet

Colorful fruits and vegetables

Whole grains and nuts

Legumes (beans)

Olive oil as the main source of fat calories

Seafood

Very little meat

Cheese in moderation

Red wine with meals

The men taking part in the Seven Countries Study were surveyed at five-year intervals, and in 1984 a fifteen-year recap revealed that Cretans had lower rates of heart disease and death than even the Japanese, who had low rates of heart disease and death when compared to the people in the United States, Finland, Yugoslavia, the Netherlands, and Italy.[1]

The Seven Countries Study demonstrated a close association between high blood levels of cholesterol, dietary intake of *saturated fat* (fats that are solid at room temperature, found mainly in meat and dairy products), heart disease, and premature death. But as so often happens, people took away the wrong message from this finding. Fats suddenly became anathema, even though it was only saturated fats that were implicated in bad outcomes. Unfortunately, all fats got tarred with the same brush.

Lost in the rush to condemn fats was the fantastic benefit that occurred with the ingestion of the *monounsaturated fats* found in olive oil and the *omega-3 fats* found in fish. The prestigious American Heart Association (AHA) for years preached the gospel of low-fat diets, calling the restriction of fat intake the "cornerstone" of its dietary recommendations. What led to this basic misconception about dietary fat?

In the 1950s there was little understanding or knowledge of the lipoproteins, the specialized proteins that transport the various blood fats. Only total cholesterol was measured, and studies examined the effects of different fats on total cholesterol. *Polyunsaturated fats* (fats that are liquid at room temperature, derived mainly from plant sources) were found to lower total cholesterol, but monounsaturated fats had no effect. We now know that both kinds of fats lower the bad LDL cholesterol when they are substituted for saturated fats, but only monounsaturated fats raise the good HDL cholesterol. The two effects of monounsaturated fats (raising HDL cholesterol, lowering LDL cholesterol) cancelled each other out when it came to the total cholesterol level. Since polyunsaturated fats alone lowered total cholesterol, they were touted as being the healthiest kind of fats. But in 1986, another analysis of the Seven Countries Study showed that the ratio of monounsaturated to saturated fat was the best predictor of health.[2] Those people who had the highest intake of monounsaturated fats and the lowest intake of saturated fats had the lowest mortality rates as well as the lowest rates of both heart disease *and* cancer.

But the Seven Countries Study was an observational study, not a randomized, controlled trial. Observational studies may tell us about *association* but they cannot prove *causation*. In other words, something other than the Mediterranean diet may have been the cause of the low rates of heart disease in Crete. Maybe the real reason that Cretan men did so well was all the exercise they got, or the naps they took after lunch, or their closeness to nature in an area of the world almost unmatched for beauty. The Seven Countries Study could not tell us for certain that their diet was the reason for their good health and longevity. However, it did prompt researchers to undertake studies that would prove or disprove what came to be known as the *diet-heart hypothesis*. In simple terms, the diet-heart hypothesis proposed a causal relationship among saturated fat and the cholesterol content of a diet, the blood level of cholesterol, and the development of ASCVD.

Dietary Trials to Prove the Diet-Heart Hypothesis

Early attempts at dietary trials to reduce the risk of cardiac events were not successful. Three studies involving almost 1,300 men with heart disease in England,

Norway, and Australia used diets with high ratios of polyunsaturated to saturated fats, limited dietary cholesterol, and low levels of monounsaturated fat. The studies were carried out in the 1960s and 1970s, long before statins were in use. The trials lasted five years, and despite achieving lower cholesterol levels, people on the experimental diet did not do any better than their counterparts did on the control diet.

In the Australian study, only total mortality was reported, and it was actually slightly higher in the group on the experimental diet than in the control group. There was no difference at all between the experimental and control groups in the UK study for both mortality and morbidity. The Norwegian trial saw a borderline significant difference between groups only in the composite end point of cardiac death and nonfatal heart attack.[3] But you'll notice that these studies did not utilize the Mediterranean diet as the experimental diet. That was almost certainly why they failed to bring about any beneficial effect on cardiovascular event rates.

The Lyon Diet Heart Study

During the 1980s, new dietary trials were undertaken. These were strongly influenced by Dr. Keys's work and had more positive results than the earlier clinical research. The best known of these was the Lyon Diet Heart Study: a randomized secondary prevention trial designed to test the hypothesis that a Mediterranean-type diet would reduce the rate of cardiac events in people who'd suffered heart attacks. The control group in this study was put on a "prudent" Western-type diet. The experimental diet was very high in a plant-derived omega-3 polyunsaturated fat, linolenic acid, incorporated in a margarine that replaced cream and butter. Compared to the prudent diet, the experimental diet had more bread, green and root vegetables, and poultry and less beef, lamb, and pork. Fruit was eaten every day. The study was single-blind, not double-blind, because the subjects obviously knew which diet they were on. However, the investigators who adjudicated the clinical end points did not know which diet was being followed by the people who had end point events.

The patients were recruited after a first heart attack, were under seventy years of age, and were stable healthwise. The recruitment period went from March 1988 until March 1992. A total of 302 experimental and 303 control group subjects were randomized into the study in such a way as to ensure that both groups had similar risk factor profiles. The average follow-up period was forty-six months per patient. Taking part in the final study visit were 219 people in the experimental group and 204 people in the control group. The results were unlike anything seen in prior diet trials: 19 people on the control diet suffered cardiac death (a rate of 1.37 per one hundred person years) compared to 6 people on the Mediterranean diet (a rate of 0.41 per one hundred person years); 25 people on the control diet had a nonfatal heart attack (a rate of 2.7 per one hundred person years) compared to 8 people on the Mediterranean diet (a rate of 0.83 per 100 person years). Even all-cause mortality was reduced: 24 people in the control group versus 14 in the experimental group, or 1.74 per one hundred person years, versus 0.95 per one hundred person years. Overall, the relative risk reductions were truly amazing. There was a 56 percent reduction in the risk of death from any cause, a 65 percent reduction in the risk of cardiac death, and a 70 percent reduction in the risk of heart attack. There was even a 61 percent reduction in the risk of developing cancer. All of these results were statistically significant and occurred despite the fact that the LDL cholesterol levels did not differ significantly between the two groups. At the final study visit, the subjects on the Mediterranean and control diets had average LDL cholesterol values of 161 and 164 respectively.[4] In other words, you can lower the risk of cardiac events in people who've already had a heart attack *without* lowering their LDL cholesterol levels.

That is not the kind of information Big Pharma wants you to have. It might make you look with a jaundiced eye at the statin medicine that is causing you to walk around aching all the time.

If you check out the AHA website write-up of this study, the reaction to the results of the Lyon Diet Heart Study is tepid at best: "The results suggest that a Mediterranean-style Step I diet may help reduce recurrent events in patients with heart disease."[5] *Suggest? May* help reduce recurrent events? Could this have anything to do with the billions of dollars that the AHA obtains from industry, particularly Big Pharma?

At its annual meeting and in its journal, *Circulation,*

the American Heart Association pushes statin therapy with all its attendant dangers on ever greater numbers of people. It is hard to escape the conclusion that the organization deliberately downplays the benefits of a diet that has been proven to lower the risk of heart disease. A diet that has no side effects except to make you healthier, but a diet that doesn't make Big Pharma any profits.

More Proof of the Benefits of the Mediterranean Diet

The results of the Lyon Diet Heart Study are reinforced by an observational study undertaken more recently. An article published in the *Archives of Internal Medicine* in 2007[6] reported on a study of 214,284 men and 166,012 women who participated in a clinical trial researching the effect of the Mediterranean diet on mortality between 1995 and 2005. All were healthy and free of cancer and heart disease at the beginning of the study. Men whose diet conformed most to the Mediterranean diet lowered their risk of death from any cause by 23 percent, death from cancer by 21 percent, and death from cardiovascular disease by 24 percent when compared to those whose diet conformed least. The comparable numbers for women were 22 percent, 14 percent, and 21 percent. The authors concluded that the more closely participants followed the Mediterranean dietary pattern, the greater was their reduction in all-cause mortality, including mortality due to cancer and CVD.

Why the Mediterranean Diet Works

Several excellent studies elucidate the mechanisms by which the Mediterranean diet confers protection against chronic disease. There is not just one beneficial result of the Mediterranean diet. As study after study has shown, adhering to the Mediterranean diet has multiple beneficial effects on risk factors for atherosclerotic cardiovascular disease. Controlling risk factors—or, better yet, preventing them altogether—is the best way to lower the toll of suffering and death from heart disease, because there is no cure for ASCVD. All the stents, bypass operations, and medications thrown at this condition can only control its symptoms or slow its progression. There is no magic Roto-Rooter that can dissolve or suck out plaque. So how well does the Mediterranean diet do at controlling risk factors?

An elegant study published in the *Archives of Internal Medicine* in 2000[7] randomized ten men and thirteen women with high blood pressure to two different diets—each for six months—after which the subjects then crossed over to the other diet. One diet was enriched with *oleic acid,* the monounsaturated fatty acid (MUFA) found in olive oil. During this part of the study, the subjects received extra-virgin olive oil. The other diet was enriched with polyunsaturated fatty acids (PUFA) in the form of sunflower oil.

Olive oil differs from sunflower oil not only in its fatty acid content but also in other respects. It is richer in *polyphenols* (a class of phytochemicals: chemicals that evolved in plants to protect them from predators), which have anti-inflammatory and antioxidant properties. It is the oxidized form of LDL cholesterol that gets into the arterial wall and spurs plaque formation, and plaques with more inflammation are more likely to rupture and cause heart attacks. In addition, oxidized LDL cholesterol impairs the ability of arteries to relax and dilate. Stiffer arteries lead to increased blood pressure. So polyphenols found in olive oil inhibit the process of oxidation, lending a protective effect. Sunflower oil does not contain any antioxidant polyphenols, whereas 10 grams of extra-virgin olive oil has as many as 5 milligrams of them. Sunflower oil is also made up predominantly of omega-6 fatty acids, and a high intake of omega-6 fatty acids is thought to increase inflammation.

So what did the researchers observe in these people with high blood pressure? Systolic pressure (the higher of the two blood pressure numbers) was significantly lower on the MUFA diet compared to the PUFA diet (127 millimeters of mercury, or mmHg, versus 135 mmHg). Diastolic pressure (the lower blood pressure number) was also significantly lower (84 versus 90). The daily dosage of antihypertensive medicine needed to control blood pressure was also reduced by 48 percent on the MUFA diet but by only 4 percent on the PUFA diet, another statistically significant difference. This blood-pressure-lowering effect of the main fat in the Mediterranean diet is one explanation for its ability to combat ASCVD. But there are others.

Diet Can Lower Bad Cholesterol by the Same Amount as a Statin Can

What about the effect of the Mediterranean diet on LDL cholesterol level and C-reactive protein blood levels? Big Pharma would like you to think that only taking statin medicines will lower your LDL cholesterol by an appreciable amount. But this is refuted by a study published in the *Journal of the American Medical Association* (*JAMA*) in 2003.[8] Forty-six healthy adult Canadians with high cholesterol (25 men and 21 postmenopausal women) and an average age of fifty-nine years were randomly assigned to undergo one of three dietary interventions in an outpatient setting for one month. The three interventions were a diet very low in saturated fat (the control diet), the same diet plus 20 milligrams of lovastatin per day, or a diet high in plant sterols, soy protein, soluble fiber, and almonds (the Portfolio diet). Both plant sterols and soluble fiber decrease cholesterol levels: plant sterols by inhibiting the absorption of cholesterol and soluble fiber by increasing the excretion of cholesterol in the bowel. Soy protein reduces the synthesis of cholesterol in the liver and may increase the organ's uptake of cholesterol, thereby lowering the amount of cholesterol in the blood by yet another mechanism.

The main outcomes measured were lipid and CRP levels, blood pressure, and body weight. At the end of four weeks, the control diet group had an 8 percent drop in LDL cholesterol; the statin diet group, a 30.9 percent drop in LDL cholesterol; and the Portfolio diet group, a 28.6 percent drop in LDL cholesterol. There was no significant difference in the statin and Portfolio diet groups with respect to lowering LDL cholesterol. In other words, you can drop your bad cholesterol the same amount with diet as you can with a statin.

If you look at the ratio of LDL cholesterol to HDL cholesterol (you want that to drop; in other words, you want LDL cholesterol lower and HDL cholesterol higher), the diet that was very low in saturated fat actually caused a 3 percent *increase* in this ratio, although this was not statistically significant, while the ratio dropped 28.4 percent in the statin diet group and 23.5 percent in the Portfolio diet group.

CRP dropped 10 percent in the control diet group, 33.3 percent in the statin diet group, and 28.2 percent in the Portfolio diet group. Remember, the reductions in blood cholesterol levels in both the statin diet group and the Portfolio diet group were statistically greater than the changes in the control diet group, but there was no significant difference between the reduction achieved in the statin group compared to the Portfolio diet group. The same thing held true for the CRP reductions. Both the statin and Portfolio diet groups achieved statistically significant greater reductions than the control diet group, but there was no significant difference between the statin group and the Portfolio diet group in CRP reduction. Women achieved the same benefit as men.

The authors calculated the coronary heart disease risk and found it to be similarly reduced in the statin and Portfolio diet groups (25.8 percent and 24.9 percent, respectively) and significantly greater than the

3 percent reduction in the control group. The bottom line is that the Portfolio diet was every bit as good as statin therapy plus a low saturated fat diet in lowering LDL cholesterol and CRP.

Unlike the JUPITER trial, this study did not receive reams of publicity in the medical and lay presses. Did this have anything to do with the fact that if more people knew about the results, Big Pharma's profits might be affected?

A much larger study of the effects of the Mediterranean diet on risk factors for heart disease was reported in the *Annals of Internal Medicine* in 2006.[9] In this trial, 772 healthy people between the ages of fifty-five and eighty—without symptoms of heart disease but considered at risk—were randomized to either a low-fat diet recommended by the American Heart Association or one of two Mediterranean diets. The study took place in ten medical centers in Spain. Participants had to meet at least one of two criteria: (1) a diagnosis of adult-onset diabetes or (2) three or more risk factors for ASCVD such as current smoking, high blood pressure, high LDL cholesterol, low HDL cholesterol, being overweight, or a family history of premature coronary heart disease (CHD). Those assigned to the Mediterranean diets were given nutritional education and either 1 liter of extra-virgin olive oil a week or 30 grams per day of walnuts, hazelnuts, and almonds. The outcomes were measured at three months, and included body weight, body mass index (BMI), waist measurement, blood pressure, blood lipids, blood sugar, and inflammatory markers.

However, the entire study, which involves about nine thousand people and which goes by the acronym PREDIMED, standing for the Prevención con Dieta Mediterránea study, was projected to last until 2011. The primary end point was to be the composite of cardiovascular death, nonfatal heart attack, and nonfatal stroke. This article just reported data obtained after three months on the diets, in a subset of the entire study population.

Body weight, BMI, and waist measurements declined slightly in all three groups but were not significantly different among the groups. Compared to the people assigned to the low-fat diet, those on either of the two Mediterranean diets exhibited significantly reduced systolic and diastolic blood pressures and blood sugar levels. They also decreased their ratio of total cholesterol to HDL cholesterol and increased their HDL cholesterol level. Total cholesterol and triglyceride levels decreased only in the Mediterranean diet with nuts group. The Mediterranean diet groups also demonstrated improved sensitivity to insulin, the hormone that regulates blood sugar levels, a beneficial finding in that resistance to the action of insulin is associated with many adverse cardiovascular effects.

The researchers also found interesting changes in various inflammatory markers. CRP levels decreased only in people who were on the Mediterranean diet supplemented with olive oil. There were no significant changes in CRP in people on the low-fat diet or the nut-supplemented Mediterranean diet. The average decrease in CRP in the olive oil–supplemented group was an impressive 0.54. Interestingly, the study also looked at some other inflammatory markers and found that all decreased significantly in people on either Mediterranean diet, and increased significantly in the low-fat diet group. In other words, the low-fat diet preached by the AHA for years actually increased the amount of inflammation in the body, thereby increasing the likelihood of atherosclerosis!

And despite the fact that the Mediterranean diets were high-fat diets, and many of the people in the study were diabetic or obese, there was no weight gain on average when these diets were supplemented with sizeable amounts of unsaturated fats in the form of nuts and olive oil. In fact, there was slight weight loss. The study was supported by a grant from the Spanish Ministry of Health. Other sponsorship was provided by the Fundacion Patrimonio Comunal Olivarero (a nonprofit organization under the Spanish Ministry of the Environment and Rural and Marine Affairs, which promotes olive oil consumption), Oleícola Hojiblanca SA (an olive oil cooperative), the California Walnut Commission, Borges S.A. (an olive oil and nut supplier), and Morella Nuts S.A., which donated the olive oil, walnuts, almonds, and hazelnuts, respectively, in the study. But the funding sources "had no role in the design, collection, analysis, or interpretation of the data."

Contrast this with how the JUPITER trial was funded and run. And contrast the hoopla surrounding the publication of the JUPITER trial with the yawn that greeted the publication of this important diet study.

Antioxidant Effect of the Mediterranean Diet

The Mediterranean diet is rich in antioxidants, so it stands to reason that you could measure whether it had an effect on the oxidation of lipoproteins. A subset of the people in the PREDIMED trial, 210 women and 162 men, had their oxidized LDL cholesterols measured after three months on either the control diet or the Mediterranean diets.[10] The authors pointed out that current evidence implicated "oxidative damage" as a promoter of changes that occur in many diseases, including CHD and cancer, as well as certain neurodegenerative disorders and in aging.

Earlier observational studies had shown that adhering to a Mediterranean diet was associated with lower levels of plasma oxidized LDL cholesterol (Ox-LDL) in the blood, but prior to this study, no randomized controlled intervention study had assessed the ability of the Mediterranean diet to lower Ox-LDL. After three months, both the olive oil–supplemented and nut-supplemented Mediterranean diet groups had statistically significant drops in their Ox-LDL levels compared to the control diet group, decreasing by 10.6 U/L and 7.3 U/L, respectively; there was no significant decrease in the control group. (U/L stands for units per liter.)The authors concluded that the study's results "provide further evidence to recommend the traditional Mediterranean diet as a useful tool against risk factors for CHD."

Weight Loss and the Mediterranean Diet

Finally, let's look at what is probably the hardest AS-CVD risk factor to modify: obesity. For decades in the United States, the scientific establishment preached the low-fat-diet gospel as the best way to lose weight. Over those same decades, the rates of overweight and obesity skyrocketed. Low-fat diets were clearly not working, or people just were not following them. (We'll get to why that might be a bit later.) So if low-fat diets don't work, what does?

The late Dr. Robert Atkins would have you believe that a high-fat diet works not only to make you lose weight but to prevent heart disease. The fact that he himself died of a sudden cardiac arrest is therefore disconcerting, since he followed his own Atkins diet.

So what happened when the Mediterranean diet went head-to-head with a low-fat diet and a low-carbohydrate diet?[11] Unlike many short-term diet trials, this was a two-year study in which 322 moderately obese people were randomized to one of three diets: low fat, restricted calorie; Mediterranean, restricted calorie; or low carbohydrate, nonrestricted calorie. There were 277 men and only 45 women in the trial. The rates of adherence to a study diet were quite good: 95.4 percent at one year and 84.6 percent at two years. The people in the clinical trial were between the ages of forty and sixty-five, and had either (1) a BMI of at least 27 (in other words, they were overweight or obese), (2) diabetes, or (3) CHD regardless of age and BMI. The low-fat, restricted-calorie diet was based on American Heart Association guidelines, with the aim of restricting calories to 1,500 a day in women and 1,800 a day in men. Thirty percent of calories came from fat, 10 percent of calories were derived from saturated fat, and cholesterol intake was limited to 300 milligrams a day. Participants were counseled to eat low-fat grains, vegetables, fruits, and legumes, and to limit their intake of additional fats, sweets, and high-fat snacks.

The Mediterranean diet was a moderate-fat, restricted-calorie diet rich in vegetables and low in red meat, with poultry and fish replacing beef and lamb. The calorie restriction in this diet was the same as in the low-fat diet, with a goal of no more than 35 percent of calories from fat. The main sources of added fat were olive oil and nuts.

The low-carbohydrate, nonrestricted-calorie diet aimed to limit carbohydrate intake to 20 grams a day for a two-month induction period, with a gradual increase to a maximum of 120 grams a day to maintain weight loss. The intakes of total calories, protein, and fat were unrestricted. However, in the Atkins diet group, the participants were advised to avoid *trans fats* and to choose vegetarian sources of fat and protein. Trans fats, also called partially hydrogenated vegetable oils, are manufactured fats found in many processed foods, including most snack foods and fast foods, such as McDonald's French fries. Trans fats raise LDL cholesterol and lower HDL cholesterol. It would be difficult to find a more harmful fat if you tried. And yet any call to remove trans fats from food or restaurant menus is met with fierce opposition from food manufacturing companies anxious to protect their profits. And don't be fooled by food labels: the label can read 0 trans fat as long as there is less than 500 milligrams per serving. So read the list of ingredients, and if you see "partially hydrogenated vegetable oil," don't buy it. It contains trans fats.

The people in the study were weighed every month. The weight loss after twenty-four months for the entire study population averaged 6.4 pounds in the low-fat-diet group, 9.7 pounds in the Mediterranean diet group, and 10.4 pounds in the low-carbohydrate group. There were interesting differences in the results when you compared men to women. The men's average weight loss in the three diets was 7.5 pounds, 8.8 pounds, and 10.8 pounds, respectively. For women, the comparable numbers were an average weight loss of 0.22 pounds, 13.7 pounds, and 5.3 pounds, respectively. So for women who want to lose weight, the Mediterranean diet was the clear winner. But no matter how you sliced it, low-fat diets were not nearly as effective for weight loss as either the Mediterranean diet or the low-carbohydrate diet.

The Mediterranean diet group had the highest ratio of monounsaturated fat to saturated fat, and the highest amount of dietary fiber. LDL cholesterol levels fell most in the Mediterranean diet group and fell least in the low-fat diet group, but the differences among the groups were not statistically significant. HDL cholesterol rose in all groups—as would be expected with weight loss—but rose most in the low-carbohydrate group, and triglycerides fell only slightly in the low-fat diet but fell significantly in the Mediterranean and low-carbohydrate diet groups. The level of hsCRP decreased significantly in the Mediterranean diet group and the low-carbohydrate group, with no significant difference between these two groups with respect to hsCRP.

Among the thirty-six people with diabetes in this trial, changes in fasting blood sugar and insulin levels were more favorable among those assigned to the Mediterranean diet than among those on the low-fat diet.

In summary, the studies that compared the Mediterranean diet to the "prudent" low-fat diet pushed on people for years had unequivocal results: the Mediterranean diet improves risk factors, while the so-called prudent diet actually makes some risk factors worse. So the adherents of the low-fat-diet gospel have been shown to be flat-out wrong. What's more, they may have contributed to the problem. Dr. Sylvan Weinberg wrote an article in the *Journal of the American College of Cardiology* in 2004[12] in which he concluded that low-fat, high-carbohydrate diets "may have played an unintended role" in the epidemics of obesity, diabetes, and blood lipid abnormalities that we are now experiencing. He also pointed out that such a diet should no longer be "defended by appeal to the authority of prestigious medical organizations."

I would add that the diet cannot be defended, particularly when these "prestigious medical organizations" such as the American Heart Association are beholden to their supporters in Big Pharma and the food-producing conglomerates.

Debunking Some Other Diet Myths

Before we leave the subject of diets, I'd like to correct a common misconception: that eating eggs and shellfish, which contain cholesterol, raises your cholesterol levels and increases your risk of heart disease. My patients are amazed and often delighted when I tell them that they can eat all the shrimp, lobster, crab, and eggs they want. Why? Because eating pure cholesterol doesn't raise your cholesterol to any appreciable degree. Eating *saturated fat* raises your cholesterol levels; specifically, your LDL and HDL cholesterol.

Egg yolks, where all the cholesterol is found, contain about 200 milligrams of cholesterol, 1.6 grams of saturated fat (about 8 percent of the recommended daily intake), 2 grams of monounsaturated fat, and a healthy serving of vitamins and minerals. Four large shrimp contain 0.1 grams of saturated fat and 43 milligrams of cholesterol. A whole cup of cooked lobster meat contains 0.2 grams of saturated fat and 104 milligrams of cholesterol.[13]

All of these foods also supply complete protein and may definitely be part of a heart-healthy diet. Other seafoods, especially oily fish such as salmon, trout, sardines, and anchovies, should be eaten at least twice a week to ensure that you are getting enough of the anti-inflammatory, triglyceride-lowering omega-3 fatty acids.

As a recent review concluded, the available evidence indicates that "dietary cholesterol makes no significant contribution to atherosclerosis and risk of cardiovascular disease."[14] The author of this review is employed by the Egg Nutrition Center, so it's likely that he's not unbiased about eggs. But other studies have looked at egg consumption and have reached similar conclusions. The bottom line is that you can eat eggs, lobster, shrimp, and crabs to your heart's content and not worry about your cholesterol levels.

All of the foregoing should have convinced you that the plant-based Mediterranean diet is far more effective than the low-fat diet as a way to lower ASCVD risk. But the story of diet involves more than just the amounts of fats, proteins, and carbohydrates in what we eat. Over the course of the last half century or so, what we eat has gone from food largely produced by Mother Nature to things largely *manufactured* by giant corporations. I call them "things" because the end result of industry tinkering is often a "product" that is almost unrecognizable as food; a product, moreover, that has been highly processed and refined and then "fortified" with some, but by no means all, of the nutrients that were there before manufacturers got their hands on it. I tell my patients that if they are really serious about their health, they will eat foods that have been monkeyed with by human beings as little as possible.

Just as Big Pharma has perverted medical science and medical practice, Big Agribusiness (Big Ag) has perverted the eating habits of the United States, other industrialized nations, and, to a greater extent every day, the so-called developing world. Michael Pollan, in his books *The Omnivore's Dilemma* and *In Defense of Food*, has written on this subject far more comprehensively than I ever could. The end result has been widespread adulteration of meats, farmed fish, vegetables, and fruits with hormones, antibiotics, pesticides, and additives to prolong shelf life. At the same time, the living conditions of the animals that wind up on our tables are hellish to an extent that even Dante's *Inferno* fails to imagine. Animals are subjected to bioengineering so that they mature in a shorter time and yield increased meat for the same amount of feed. This often involves adding growth hormones to their food. They are kept in such cramped conditions that infectious diseases would be rampant were they not fed daily doses of antibiotics. For example, chickens raised for egg laying are kept in stacks of cages so small (sixty-seven square inches of floor space, in stacks three to nine tiers high)[15] that they develop deformities from rubbing against their cages and infections from weakened immune systems. Many food scientists and physicians are convinced that the practice of adding antibiotics to animal feed has facilitated the emergence of the "super bugs": bacteria resistant to multiple antibiotics.

The FDA, which tiptoes around Big Pharma, has been ineffective in curbing Big Ag's widespread use of antibiotics. Granted, the FDA has been thwarted in the past by Big Ag and its lobbyists, who have the ear of Congress and the bucks to buy influence. Another article in the *New York Times*, "Antibiotics in Animals Need Limits, FDA Says," by Gardiner Harris on June 28, 2010, noted that federal regulators have tried to ban the use of antibiotics in the water and food given to cattle and other animals to help prevent the emergence of dangerous bacteria but have been unsuccessful for more than thirty years. This lack of success is because Congress, at the behest of agricultural lobbyists, has kept the FDA from acting. Or, as Mr. Harris puts it: "In the battle between public health and agriculture, the guys with the cowboy hats generally win."

The upshot is that our food supply is degraded and potentially dangerous, while the agency charged with protecting it is asleep on the job. Nor is that the only way in which our current diets are harmful. In 2010 Dr. Anthony DeMaria, editor in chief of the *Journal of the American College of Cardiology*, wrote an editorial in which he cited Michael Pollan's books.

Pollan "argued that nutrition science had succeeded in breaking down plants and animals into their component parts and then reassembling them into high-value-added food systems that were neither high value nor, in fact, actually food. The fabricated products were often high calorie, toxic, or contaminated with antibiotics or hormones . . ."

Dr. DeMaria goes on to discuss the evolution of our concepts regarding food and nutrition science, as explained by Pollan. He writes about the proclamation by the FDA that processed foods could not be classified as imitations if they were nutritionally equivalent to food that had not been processed. This led to the "industrialization" of food, and what the food industry emphasized was not the whole food but the nutrients it contained. The outcome of all this tinkering with food was a Western diet that contained not natural food but fabricated foods, based more on seeds than whole plants, with the addition of preservatives and additives, and for the most part deficient in phytochemicals, fiber, and antioxidants.[16]

In summary, as Dr. DeMaria notes, Pollan recommends, only partially tongue in cheek, "eat food, not too much, mostly plants."[17] I would add: and douse those plants with a healthy helping of olive oil. (For a sampling of heart-healthy recipes inspired by the Mediterranean diet, see chapter 10.)

The Mediterranean diet has science to back it up, incorporates real food that tastes great, and has no known adverse effects. Why would anyone in his or her right mind choose to take powerful medicines with scary side effects when a delicious diet can accomplish the same goal of lowering risk factors for heart disease?

The metaphor I use with my male patients goes like this: pretend that someone said he'd give you a free Ferrari Testarossa. The catch is that it's the *only* car you'll ever own. You can't get another one, ever. Would you put the lowest grade of gasoline from a no-name gas station in its tank? Would you buy the cheapest motor oil and then forget to have the oil changed? Would you neglect to bring it in to the mechanic for regular checkups and tune-ups? Would you let it sit in the garage and never let that gorgeous 12-cylinder engine gallop down the road? Of course you wouldn't! You'd put only the best-quality products in that baby, you'd be a fanatic about maintenance, and you'd take her out for regular spins.

So why don't you take the same kind of care of your body? It's the only one you'll ever have. You can't trade it in. The best you can do is maybe replace some parts if they wear out, or unclog some pipes. So pretend that your body is a Ferrari Testarossa, and treat it accordingly.

Men really seem to get that.

Exercise

Having beaten the diet horse practically to death, I'm now going to write just a few words about exercise. I won't bore you with all the studies that have shown that people who exercise regularly live longer, healthier lives than couch potatoes. You already know that. We *all* know that, but most of us don't act on that knowledge. I do, but not just to be healthier physically. I find that the greatest benefits of regular exercise are mental and emotional. It's the best stress reliever around. I tell my patients that if I didn't exercise, I would probably be in either our local psychiatric hospital or our local prison. There are few guarantees in life other than death and taxes, but I can guarantee you that if you exercise regularly, *you will feel better.* You'll also look better, although that's less important.

The current recommendations are that you accumulate at least 150 minutes of moderate exercise a week. An example of moderate exercise is walking at three miles an hour. It's okay to cram those 150 minutes in over the weekend, if you work full time and can't find the time to squeeze in a workout between your job, your family, and your other responsibilities. But you have to set aside the time and let nothing short of a catastrophe interfere. Rather than a pill to treat cholesterol, what I'd really love to be able to prescribe is a pill that made people crave exercise.

Other Things You Need to Do

For the rest, avoiding secondhand smoke is becoming easier as more and more states are making indoor smoking illegal. If you are addicted to nicotine, you need to get into a smoking cessation program, which can be found at almost any hospital. If your nearest hospital is too far away for easy access, I would suggest you check the American Lung Association's Freedom from Smoking program or the American Cancer Society's Fresh Start Program. The URL's for these organizations are www.lungusa.org and www.cancer.org.

It's important that you know your own level of risk for cardiovascular disease, which means seeing a physician once a year even if you are healthy, and having your blood pressure, blood sugar, and cholesterol numbers measured.

In the final analysis, *you* are responsible for making the choices that will optimize your chances of a long and healthy life.

Part 2

WHYS AND WHEREFORES OF THE STATIN ERA

Chapter 6

The Chinese Got There First: Red Rice Yeast and the Dawn of the Statin Era

R.H. is a seventy-seven-year-old retired teacher who had always been told she had very high cholesterol. Her total cholesterol was in the range of 300 whenever her blood was tested. She was overweight but did not have any diagnosed heart disease, high blood pressure, or family history of premature coronary heart disease, and she had never smoked.

At about age sixty-seven, R.H. and her husband moved to Florida, and her physician there prescribed pravastatin (Pravachol) to treat her high cholesterol. She did well for a year and then began to notice a pins and needles sensation in her feet. This worsened, and then she began experiencing severe pain and weakness in her legs. It progressed to the point where she was unable to dress herself or go to the bathroom without assistance. Her husband says, "She's not a complainer, but I would wake up, and she'd be crying in pain."

Eventually she had pain in all the muscles of her body, in addition to severe weakness. R.H. became bedridden. She was treated with painkillers, but they did nothing to relieve her distress. Her statin medicine was stopped, but her symptoms continued. Her physician referred her to a pain management program where she was treated with a Duragesic patch (the patch contains fentanyl, a powerful narcotic, which is slowly absorbed from the skin into the bloodstream) and injections of steroids, but all to no avail. She was referred to a neurologist, who hospitalized her. She had multiple diagnostic tests, which confirmed that she was suffering from severe neuropathy, mainly of the femoral nerves to the legs. She was discharged to a rehabilitation facility, where she improved somewhat with intensive physical therapy, but she remained very weak and required a wheelchair to get around.

Because of her disability, R.H. and her husband moved back to the Northeast to be closer to family. She saw another neurologist, who ordered a muscle biopsy. The results showed that she suffered from mitochondrial myopathy. He put her on amitriptyline (Elavil), an antidepressant that is sometimes used to treat neuropathy. Her pain finally resolved, and her muscle strength improved, although it took about two years for it to return to near normal. She still cannot stand for prolonged periods, and she still gets pins and needles in her feet, but she is pain free. Needless to say, she is still not taking a statin.

This woman meets the current guidelines for drug treatment of her lipid levels, but a statin caused her to suffer severe side effects, affecting both muscles and nerves, which took years to resolve. She is currently not taking any cholesterol medicines. In the spring of 2010,

R.H.'s total cholesterol was 325, her HDL cholesterol was 64, and her LDL cholesterol was 237. She has no signs or symptoms of cardiovascular disease.

———

In April 2010, if you Googled *red rice yeast*, you would come up with about 1.7 million hits. I first heard about red rice yeast from my patients. Many of them are convinced that it's safer to take so-called natural supplements than prescription medicines. They are often politely disbelieving when I tell them that "natural" remedies are made up of chemicals, just as prescription medicines are. And while I find a lot to criticize about the way the FDA operates, it does exert at least *some* control over the quality of prescription drugs sold in the United States and the introduction of new medicines. The approval of new prescription medications is a tightly regulated, cumbersome, and expensive process.

Manufacturers of herbal supplements, on the other hand, don't have to get FDA approval before marketing their products. The FDA is responsible for monitoring the safety of herbal supplements once they are sold. But often the first hint of a problem with supplements is that people start getting sick or dying from them.

Fatalities from Herbal Supplements

One result of that regrettable loophole was the outbreak of eosinophilia-mylagia syndrome (EMS) in 1989, which was traced to tryptophan supplements manufactured by a Japanese company. Tryptophan is an amino acid that was often used as a sleep aid. As reported in the *Journal of the American Medical Association* in 1990,[1] the newly recognized disorder EMS caused afflicted people to suffer severe, debilitating muscle pain. They also had high levels of certain white blood cells called eosinophils. The eosinophil count can rise in people who are having an allergic reaction. As of July 1989, a total of 1,531 cases of EMS had been reported in the United States, including twenty-seven deaths. The incidence of eosinophilia-mylagia syndrome fell markedly when the tryptophan supplements were withdrawn from the market.

Plant-Derived Medicines

Plants have been used for medicinal purposes for thousands of years. One of the earliest cardiac medicines, digitalis, was derived from the foxglove plant (*Digitalis purpurea*). Extracts of willow bark were used for centuries in China, Greece, North America, and Europe to fight fever and inflammation. The active ingredient in willow bark, salicin, is similar to the active ingredient in aspirin: acetylsalicylic acid.

Red rice yeast has been consumed for centuries in China. It is made by fermenting a yeast called *Monascus pupureus* over red rice. Since around AD 800, Chinese herbalists have prescribed it for ailments ranging from digestive problems to circulatory complaints. Red rice yeast has also been used as a textile dye and in the making of wine and Peking duck. It goes by various names, including *hong qu, xuezhikang,* and *hung chu.* The trade name for one of the most common preparations of red rice yeast is Cholestin.

Over the last several decades, red rice yeast preparations have been prescribed to lower cholesterol. The reason they lower cholesterol is due at least partially to a compound they contain called monacolin K, which is identical chemically to lovastatin (Mevacor), the first FDA-approved statin medication.

In 1815 the French chemist M. E. Chevreul was the first scientist to isolate cholesterol. He found it in human gallstones, hardened nuggets of cholesterol that form mainly in the gallbladder, and named it cholesterine. The manufacture of cholesterol by the body is a complex process involving more than thirty enzymes. Cholesterol is produced by multiple organs, including the liver, intestines, and reproductive glands. An early step in cholesterol synthesis requires the action of the enzyme HMG-CoA reductase; when this enzyme is inhibited, cholesterol synthesis is blocked, and cholesterol levels drop.

Clinical trials to look at the effect of red rice yeast on cholesterol levels in the blood were undertaken during the 1990s in the United States and elsewhere. These studies showed that red rice yeast was effective in lowering total cholesterol and LDL cholesterol by about 15 percent to 20 percent.

In 2007 a study that examined the effect of red rice yeast on reducing the risk of nonfatal heart attacks and death due to heart disease in a group of Chinese diabetics with known heart disease was published in

the *Journal of Cardiovascular Physiology*.[2] This study
enrolled 591 diabetics, 306 of whom were treated with
the red rice yeast preparation called *xuezhikang,* an extract of Cholestin, and 285 received a placebo. During
an average of four years of follow-up, compared to the
people on placebo, the relative risk of a nonfatal heart
attack was reduced by 63.8 percent, the relative risk of
a fatal heart attack was reduced by 58.5 percent, and
the relative risk of death due to coronary heart disease
(CHD) was reduced by 53.4 percent in those treated
with red rice yeast.

The FDA got into the act when regulators there re-
alized that one of the ingredients of red rice yeast was
chemically indistinguishable from lovastatin. The
federal agency's position is that since red rice yeast
contains lovastatin, it is a drug and thus subject to government regulation. In 1998 the FDA banned the sale
of red rice yeast extracts that contained monacolin,
which is just another name for lovastatin. On August 9,
2007, the FDA released the following warning letter[3] to
consumers of red rice yeast products:

> The products may contain an unauthorized
> drug that could be harmful to health . . . The
> potentially harmful products . . . contain lov-
> astatin, the active pharmaceutical ingredient
> in Mevacor, a prescription drug approved for
> marketing in the United States as a treatment
> for high cholesterol . . . These red yeast rice
> products are a threat to health because the pos-
> sibility exists that lovastatin can cause severe

muscle problems leading to kidney impairment. This risk is greater in patients who take higher doses of lovastatin or who take lovastatin and other medicines that increase the risk of muscle adverse reactions. These medicines include the antidepressant nefazodone, certain antibiotics, drugs used to treat fungal infections and HIV infections, and other cholesterol-lowering medications.

Dangers of Unregulated Products

FDA efforts to stem the sale or consumption of red rice yeast products have met with little success, and dozens of brands of red rice yeast are available. In October 2010 Dr. Ram Gordon and his colleagues in Pennsylvania published the results of a study in which they analyzed several brands of red rice yeast.[4] They examined the monacolin K, total monacolin content, and citrinin (a chemical, found in some red rice yeast preparations, that can damage the kidneys) in twelve "readily available" red rice yeast formulations. They determined that the amount of monacolin K varied from 0.10 milligrams per capsule to 10.9 milligrams per capsule. More worrisome was the fact that four of these products were found to have citrinin, in concentrations varying from 24 to 189 parts per million.

So when you buy over-the-counter red rice yeast, you typically have no idea of the potency of the preparation or whether or not it contains other chemicals that are potentially harmful.

Drug Companies Enter the Market

Once scientists had established that HMG-CoA reductase was necessary for the body to make cholesterol, the race was on to discover drugs that would inhibit this enzyme. Starting in 1976, the pharmaceutical giant Merck & Co. became interested in developing an HMG-CoA reductase inhibitor. Its scientists replicated the work of two Japanese researchers, Drs. Akira Endo and Masao Kuroda, who'd isolated a substance they called mevastatin from a mold: *Penicillium citrinum*. This compound, although it lowered cholesterol, had multiple side effects and was not given to patients. Based on their work, Merck scientists isolated a compound they called lovastatin from the fungus *Aspergillus terreus*. After studies showed that lovastatin was very effective in lowering the levels of total cholesterol and LDL cholesterol, the company applied to the FDA, which approved its sale in the United States in August 1987. The drug, named Mevacor, was indicated to treat people with elevated levels of total and LDL cholesterol when dietary changes were insufficient to bring them down to healthy levels.

Over the next decade or so, the FDA granted approval for six other statin medicines: pravastatin (trade name, Pravachol), simvastatin (Zocor), fluvastatin (Lescol), atorvastatin (Lipitor), and rosuvastatin (Crestor). Cerivastatin (Baycol) was approved in 1997 but was disapproved and withdrawn from the market by the FDA in 2001, as mentioned in chapter 2.

The statin genie was out of the bottle. Big Pharma was not slow to recognize the enormous moneymaking potential of these drugs, particularly if, in addition to lowering cholesterol, statins could be shown to lower the risk of heart disease, the number one killer in the world except in sub-Saharan Africa. The race was on to produce evidence that statins could lower heart disease risk, and medical research underwent a sea change. The story of how Big Pharma came to dominate clinical research is recounted in the next chapter.

— Chapter 7 —

Big Pharma, the FDA, and the Medical Profession: An Unholy, Very Lucrative Alliance

Like all physicians, I've had interactions with pharmaceutical companies. Shortly after I went into private practice in Rhode Island in 1977, I received a telephone call from a drug company representative. He offered me an all-expense-paid weeklong trip to Germany to attend a medical conference. I was taken aback, knowing that the cost of such a trip would run to thousands of dollars. I replied that I was in solo private practice and was the single mother of three young children, so I was not free to attend. I also felt this was a not-so-subtle attempt to make me feel beholden, to influence me in favor of his company's medications.

Over the years, I have met with drug company representatives in my office because they can provide free samples of whatever drugs they are promoting, and sometimes my getting free samples is the only way that some of my patients can afford their medications. I've also attended drug company dinners where a paid expert lectures on one drug or another. Spouses used to be welcomed at these dinners, and my husband attended a few. But with increasing attention focused upon the ethics of drug company–physician interactions, medical organizations and the pharmaceutical industry agreed that it was no longer appropriate for spouses to be included in these venues.

After many years in private practice, I was asked by the CEO of my hospital to set up and direct a Women's Cardiac Center, so, since 2002, I have been a salaried hospital employee. Despite the fact that my office door now says Women's Cardiac Center, many of my male patients from my former practice still come to me, and many of the women patients I see want me to take care of their male relatives. Throughout my time in Rhode Island, I have been on the clinical faculty at Brown University's medical school. I have supervised and taught scores of medical students, interns, residents, and fellows, a part of my job that I find very rewarding. I enjoy both bedside teaching and lecturing. And being exposed to bright young physicians on a daily basis spurs me to always keep up with the latest research in my chosen field of cardiology.

About the time my first book came out in 2004 (*How to Keep from Breaking Your Heart: What Every Woman Needs to Know About Cardiovascular Disease*), a Pfizer representative whom I'd gotten to know over several years asked me if I would be interested in becoming a speaker for Pfizer, specifically on Lipitor, the company's premier statin drug. I told her that I would be happy to speak about gender-specific aspects of heart disease in women, but that I wasn't interested in just getting up in front of a bunch of doctors and plugging one or another of Pfizer's medicines. She assured me that my chosen topic would be fine, and I went off for a two-day course in New York, where various physicians, scientists, and Pfizer officials lectured on being effective speakers, demonstrated the slide sets to use, and took us through the FDA-approved indications for Lipitor.

I then made up my own slide sets on heart disease in women and began to be invited to give Pfizer-sponsored dinner talks in restaurants and Pfizer-sponsored lectures at hospitals in New England and the surrounding states. (Most, if not all, hospitals provide opportunities for their staff physicians to keep up with continuing medical education requirements by sponsoring educational lectures, called grand rounds, on the latest advances in medicine.) Pfizer paid very well: $1,000 for a lecture that didn't involve travel out of Rhode Island, and $1,500 plus travel expenses for lectures out of state. My talks on gender-specific aspects of heart disease seemed to be well received, and I felt I was educating doctors on an important subject that might be unfamiliar to them.

Despite the fact that Pfizer was sponsoring my talks, I never failed to point out that there was no evidence that Lipitor—or any statin for that matter—prevented cardiac events in women who did not have established cardiovascular disease. I mentioned the results of the ASCOT-LLA study, in which there were seventeen primary end points out of about 1,500 women in the placebo group and nineteen primary end points out of about 1,500 women in the Lipitor-treated group.

One night a regional manager attended one of my

talks—and suddenly I was no longer invited by Pfizer to give lectures.

In 2006 the Women's Cardiac Center at the Miriam Hospital was chosen to be one of the sites to participate in a large clinical trial sponsored by the National Heart, Lung, and Blood Institute (NHLBI) and by Kos Pharmaceuticals, the company that made Niaspan, a long-acting, high-dose version of the B vitamin niacin. (Kos was subsequently bought by Abbott Laboratories, which continued to cosponsor the trial.)

Niacin, in high doses, does all the right things to blood fat levels: it lowers triglycerides, lowers LDL cholesterol, and raises HDL cholesterol. The hypothesis proposed by the study designers, Drs. B. Greg Brown and William Boden, was that "extended-release niacin and simvastatin would prove superior to simvastatin alone at equivalent on-treatment LDL cholesterol levels in reducing clinical cardiovascular events in patients with established vascular disease, low HDL-C, and high triglycerides."

This trial went by the catchy name AIM-HIGH, which stands for Atherothrombosis Drug Intervention for Metabolic Syndrome with Low HDL/High Triglycerides and Its Impact on Global Health Outcomes. The AIM-HIGH trial was interested in recruiting as many women as possible. It was expected that the trial would be completed in 2012. However, the study was ended in April 2011 when the Data Monitoring and Safety Board concluded that, based on the results to date, extended-release niacin offered no benefits beyond statin therapy alone in reducing clinical events.

The AIM-HIGH trial recruited over three thousand people at ninety-eight centers around the United States and Canada. I was the principal investigator at the Women's Cardiac Center site. Every time we randomized someone into the study, and every time we saw someone for a study visit, my hospital got paid by the sponsors. None of that money came to me, nor was my salary based on the number of patients that we recruited into the trial.

Abbott Laboratories expressed interest in adding me to its speaker's bureau, and I told the company the same thing that I had told Pfizer: I would be happy to lecture about gender-specific aspects of cardiovascular disease, but not just about its products. (Abbott also sells fenofibrate, or Tricor, another lipid-lowering medicine, though not a statin. It has actions similar to niacin but works by a different mechanism.) This was satisfactory for a few years, but then Abbott decided that its speakers could use only Abbott-provided slides, at which point I told the company that I was not interested in doing this and stopped speaking at Abbott-sponsored events.

I have also on occasion been paid by the medical device companies Medtronic and Guidant Corporation to speak on gender-specific aspects of heart disease, but I neither insert medical devices myself nor teach cardiology fellows how to do these procedures. So, all in all, my interactions with the pharmaceutical/medical device companies have complied with ethical guidelines. Does this mean that I have not been influenced by these interactions? It certainly does not.

As Dana Katz, a bioethicist, and his colleagues wrote in the *American Journal of Bioethics* in 2003: "When a gift or a gesture of any size is bestowed, it imposes on the recipient a sense of indebtedness. The obligation to directly reciprocate, whether or not the recipient is directly conscious of it, tends to influence behavior."[1]

Indeed, there is an increasing body of knowledge on the ways that seemingly rational decisions can be influenced by such mundane things as receiving inexpensive gifts. Try to find a doctor's office that doesn't contain pads and pens imprinted with a pharmaceutical company's logo and the name of one of its drugs, thoughtfully provided by company representatives. Doctors bristle at the accusation that these trifles, or even the occasional free dinner-cum-lecture, can influence their prescribing habits. And on a conscious level, no doubt they are correct in saying that they are not being swayed in their prescribing decisions. But the story is not that simple. And we've known for many decades now, thanks to Sigmund Freud and others, that our subconscious plays a role in determining how we act and react. But in Freud's time, we didn't have the tools to actually investigate what aspects of brain metabolism might underlie the workings of the unconscious mind. Nowadays we do.

In 2007 the Association of American Medical Colleges held a symposium at Houston's Baylor College of Medicine entitled "The Scientific Basis of Influence and Reciprocity."[2] The seminar was designed to explore how objectivity was affected by gifts, favors, and influence. It sought to impart information about the "underlying neurobiological substrates" involved in the "process of influence and reciprocity," so that the academic community could "evaluate and manage its relationship with industry."

"Neurobiological substrates" is a fancy way of referring to changes in brain function that occur without our conscious knowledge or control. One of the participants in the symposium presented the findings of an experiment using functional MRIs (fMRIs) of the brain in people playing a "two-person trust game." Specific areas of the brain react when one receives a favor or gift from another. This research demonstrated that biologic changes occur in the brain when gifts are exchanged and that there exists "the human tendency to expect . . . that *favors given will be paid back*. In fact, the experiment suggests, but does not prove, that this process has strong automatic components that covertly influence one's decision to trust someone else."

In other words, accepting even a pen, pad, or coffee mug may generate an unconscious bias toward trusting that what a drug company representative says about his or her product is true. Big Pharma spends an estimated $30 billion a year on marketing. It is naive to believe that drug companies shell out that kind of money without proof that it works to increase sales.

But far more dangerous to our health and safety than low-cost gifts to practicing physicians is the influence that Big Pharma and medical device companies exert over academic medical centers, the supposed bastions of ethical scientific research and advanced medical care. A 2003 article in the *Journal of the American*

Medical Association reported on a survey of academic medical centers and found that almost two-thirds of them owned stock in companies that sponsored research within the same institution.[3] The authors also found a significant correlation between industry sponsorship of research and pro-industry outcomes. In other words, when a drug company was sponsoring research on one of its drugs, the study was more likely to find that the drug was beneficial than when a study was not sponsored by the company that made the drug being investigated. Industry sponsorship was also associated with restrictions on publication and data sharing.

As Marcia Angell wrote in the *Boston Review* in 2010: "The boundaries between academic medicine ... and the pharmaceutical industry have been dissolving since the 1980s, and the important differences between their missions are becoming blurred. Medical research, education, and clinical practice have suffered as a result."[4]

Medical schools and their affiliated hospitals educate each succeeding generation of doctors, employ thousands of people, are held in high esteem by the public, conduct cutting-edge research, and care for some of the sickest and poorest patients. They have a tax-exempt status that few would quibble with, given the societal benefits that they provide. The purpose of Big Pharma, on the other hand, is to maximize profits and keep their shareholders happy by paying dividends and increasing the value of their stocks. That being said, I do not deny that pharmaceutical companies have discovered many drugs that have improved and saved lives. What I want to emphasize in this chapter is the tremendous influence pharmaceutical dollars now wield over many medical schools and professional medical associations like the American Heart Association, to name just one.

As Dr. Angell noted in her article, basic research, which investigates the molecular basis of disease and tries to unlock the secrets of cellular metabolism, may not have immediate applicability to patients or lead directly to a new medicine. This is in contrast to much clinical research, the results of which often are used to justify the increased use of a drug, thereby benefiting Big Pharma's bottom line.

Basic Research and Clinical Trials

Basic research is still funded largely by the National Institutes of Health (NIH) and to a much lesser extent by charitable foundations such as the Howard Hughes Medical Institute. It was once considered the most prestigious kind of research in which to be involved. Many young physicians gravitated to the NIH, or applied for NIH grants to do this type of research. Nobel Prizes in medicine are awarded to scientists and physicians for basic research, not to those who run clinical trials.

When I was a staff associate at the NIH in the early 1970s, clinical trials were considered second-rate; they were the stepchildren of the research community. This was due partially to the fact that clinical trials in the first seven decades of the twentieth century often involved subjects who were mentally ill, imprisoned, poor, or otherwise disadvantaged. The people enrolled in these trials often did not know the purpose of the study, were not informed of the possible risks, and did not give informed consent.

The Tuskegee syphilis study is perhaps the most infamous example of such a trial. Begun in the 1930s under the aegis of the US Public Health Service, working in conjunction with the Tuskegee Institute, its purpose was to determine the effects of untreated syphilis. The study enrolled 399 mostly poor, illiterate, African-American men from Alabama who had become infected with the syphilis germ. These men had almost no access to medical care. Even after penicillin became available in the 1940s, the men in the Tuskegee study were not treated to eradicate the infection. They were allowed to die of the ravages of late-stage syphilis, including heart disease, blindness, and insanity. Even more chilling, by the end of the study, forty wives had been infected, and nineteen of their children were born with congenital syphilis.

The Tuskegee study was stopped only in 1972 when a whistle-blower, Dr. Peter Buxtun, divulged information to an Associated Press reporter, Jean Heller, and a story detailing these atrocities appeared in the *Washington Evening Star* newspaper. After a huge public outcry, the study was ended, and the surviving men were treated. In an apology to the eight remaining survivors in 1997, President Bill Clinton said, "The United States government did something that was wrong—deeply, profoundly, morally wrong. It was an outrage to our commitment to integrity and equality for all our citizens ... clearly racist."[5]

Other clinical trials included studies conducted in mental institutions where patients were infected with the influenza virus, or in prisons where inmates were injected with live cancer cells. The US government sponsored research into drugs that might compel people to tell the truth. It was not until 1965 that investigators performing clinical trials had to obtain written consent from a subject, and he or she had to be informed of the potential risks and benefits. Eventually all institutions involved in clinical research had to set up ethics boards to oversee human experimentation. These are generally called *Institutional Review Boards,* or *IRBs,* and their approval is required for any research sponsored by the NIH.

In part because of this lurid history, until the 1980s, clinical trials were considered less prestigious than basic research. But that was before Big Pharma got into the act. Nowadays, clinical trials—if they produce "positive" results—bring their principal investigators fame, wealth, interviews on network news shows, and tenured professorships. The vast majority of clinical trials are funded by pharmaceutical companies, or in some instances, such as AIM-HIGH, by the NIH in concert with a drug company.

And the rules of the game have changed. As Dr. Angell reported in her *Boston Review* article, in the past, drug companies were kept at arm's length by the medical centers that were testing their products. The research itself was often initiated by the investigator leading the study, because he or she thought that it was scientifically important. The pharmaceutical company that made the drug being studied had no part in designing the trial or analyzing the results, and it had no role in writing the journal articles that reported the study.

But thanks to the increasing dependence of academic medicine on the money generated by Big Pharma's sponsorship of clinical trials, that has all changed. Academic medical centers used to divert into research some of the money they received for taking care of patients. As reimbursements from insurers, Medicare and Medicaid have shrunk, they have turned increasingly to industry to make up the shortfall.

The result, as Dr. Angell points out, is that medical centers now defer to drug companies in ways that were unheard of a few decades ago. They have become little more than "hired hands" who supply the subjects for the trials, while they "collect data according to instructions from corporate paymasters." The sponsoring drug company may even decide whether or not the results will be submitted for publication, and sometimes, if multiple centers have taken part in the research, the principal investigators may not be allowed access to all of the data.

A glaring example of this was exposed by John Fauber writing in the *Milwaukee Journal Sentinel* on May 30, 2010.[6] The headline read, "Doctor's Role in Drug Studies Criticized." The article recounted how Dr. Richard Page, chairman of the Department of Medicine at the University of Wisconsin School of Medicine and Public Health, coauthored the report of a large international multicenter study of a new drug called dronedarone (Multaq) to treat atrial fibrillation, an abnormal heart rhythm that affects millions of people. The results of the ATHENA trial were reported in the *New England Journal of Medicine* in February 2009, and based on its findings, the FDA approved it for sale in the United States.

Dronedarone is made by Sanofi-Aventis. Not only did the pharmaceutical manufacturer fund the trial, but it also collected the raw data from the study and performed the statistical analysis "without an external audit for accuracy or completeness," according to the article in the *Milwaukee Journal Sentinel*.

In fact, although the Food and Drug Administration approved dronedarone, it refused to allow the claim, made in the *New England Journal of Medicine* article, that the drug reduced cardiovascular deaths. The FDA demanded and received access to the raw data. The study was supposed to have enrolled 4,300 patients. When this number was insufficient to show a significant benefit in reducing cardiovascular death, an additional 328 people were enrolled, and the study was extended beyond its planned cutoff date. This expanded version of the study reported that there were 90 cardiac deaths among those on placebo and 63 among those on dronedarone. But as a member of the FDA panel, Dr. Sanjay Kaul was quoted as saying: "It is not proper to change the rules in the middle of the game." In fact, it is a major no-no. The other reason to question the claim is that there was no difference in death from any cause between the two groups. Dr. Kaul concluded, "These observations raise questions about the quality of the data and ultimately the reliability of the findings."

Despite his not having seen the raw data, Dr. Page put his name on the report, thereby vouching for its accuracy. This was another of those studies that was touted as showing a statistically significant benefit of treatment on the primary end point, which was the first hospitalization for cardiovascular events or death. In the drug-treated group of about 2,300 men and women, the primary end point occurred in 31.9 percent of people, while in the similar-sized placebo-treated group, the primary end point occurred in 39.4 percent of people, for a relative risk reduction of 24 percent but an absolute risk reduction of only 7.5 percent.

About 30 percent of subjects in both groups stopped taking the assigned medicine. The people given dronedarone had a higher risk of abnormal kidney function tests, very slow heart rates, nausea, diarrhea, and rash than the people given placebo. The average follow-up was only twenty-one months, so it's conceivable that more adverse effects would have occurred had the trial lasted longer. There were potentially hundreds of millions of dollars in sales riding on the outcome of this trial. Why were the raw data kept from the principal investigators? Did Sanofi-Aventis have something to hide?

There is another reason to be concerned about the study's validity. All seven coauthors, according to Fauber's article, had financial ties to Sanofi-Aventis. Two were company employees, and the others were either paid consultants or belonged to its speakers' bureau. Could the company not find scientists without any financial ties to do this research? Did it even try?

Unanticipated Complications from Long-Term Drug Use

A classic example of side effects that become apparent only when large numbers of people take medicines for several years has come to light in the case of the heavily advertised drugs used to treat osteoporosis.

Sally Field is a talented actress, but when I see her on television touting the benefits of Boniva, I want to throw something at the screen. Boniva, the trade name for ibandronate, belongs to a class of medicines called bisphosphonates. Osteoporosis is a condition that affects mainly postmenopausal women in which bone density decreases and the risk of bone fracture increases. Our bones are constantly being remodeled, with new bone laid down and old bone resorbed. When bone resorption exceeds bone formation, osteoporosis results. The bisphosphonates work by inhibiting the resorption process.

This class of drugs is known to sometimes cause severe irritation of the esophagus, the tube leading from the mouth to the stomach. The medication must be taken on an empty stomach with 6 to 8 ounces of water, and patients are instructed to either stand or sit for thirty minutes after taking it to decrease the risk of damaging the esophagus. In addition, there have been reports of bisphosphonates leading to perforation of the gut. As you might imagine, this is a catastrophic event that can cause stubborn infections and usually requires surgical repair. Esophageal perforation can even be fatal. After repeated episodes of irritation, the tube can narrow, and these strictures can interfere with swallowing and may need to be mechanically dilated with a specialized scope that allows visualization of the narrowed area. The scope also contains a balloon which is inflated in the narrowed area to widen the stricture.

Alendronate (Fosamax) was the first bisphosphonate drug to win FDA approval in the United States, in 1995, after clinical trials showed a reduction in the risk of fractures of the hip, wrist, and vertebrae in postmenopausal women treated with alendronate compared to placebo. In one of the frequently cited studies, 994 postmenopausal women with osteoporosis who were ages forty-five to eighty were randomized to receive either alendronate or placebo and followed for three years.[7] The end points were bone mineral density and fractures. Of the women on placebo, 6.2 percent developed vertebral fractures compared to 3.2 percent of the women taking alendronate, a 48 percent relative risk reduction but a 3 percent absolute risk reduction. Bone mineral density increased 8.8 percent in the spine, 5.9 percent in the neck of the femur (the large bone in the thigh), and 7.8 percent in the trochanter, another part of the thigh bone, in women on alendronate compared to women on placebo.

After alendronate's approval by the FDA in 1995, other bisphosphonates came on the market, including risedronate (Actonel, approved in 2001), ibandronate (Boniva, approved in 2003), and zoledronic acid (Reclast, approved in 2007), a once-a-year intravenous bisphosphonate. All the other bisphosphonates are taken by mouth. Now that they have been in widespread use for over a decade, more problems are coming to light, although the pharmaceutical industry that manufactures these drugs tries to play down their danger. In fact, strange types of fractures, occurring with little to no trauma, are being reported more and more often in women taking bisphosphonates.

Fourteen articles in peer-reviewed medical journals have reported on these unusual fractures between 2005 and 2009. The fractures were felt to be a complication of bisphosphonate therapy, and yet preventing fractures from osteoporosis was the reason these medicines were prescribed in the first place!

In an attempt to limit the damage to Big Pharma's bottom line, a meta-analysis of three randomized bisphosphonate trials was published in 2010 in the *New England Journal of Medicine*.[8] The authors concluded, "There was no significant increase in risk associated with bisphosphonate use, but the study was underpowered for definitive conclusions." Can we be reassured by this statement? Most certainly not.

If you turn to the end of the article, you find out that the lead author received grants from Merck (maker of Fosamax), Novartis (maker of Reclast), and Roche (maker of Boniva). Another author received consulting and lecture fees and grant support from Merck and Novartis. Another received consulting fees from Novartis,

Roche, and more than a dozen other Big Pharma or medical device companies. Another was a full-time employee of Novartis and had an equity interest in his employer's company. Two others were full-time employees of Merck.

Do you get the impression that these were not exactly disinterested parties? And why on earth did the *New England Journal of Medicine* see fit to publish this whitewash? Any objective reader would come to the conclusion that long-term use of bisphosphonates actually weakens certain areas of bone. The FDA finally took note of all these unusual fractures and issued a statement about these reports, but said it was still investigating the link between bisphosphonates and atypical fractures.

There are other potential side effects of osteoporosis drugs. The dental literature is rife with articles about a condition called bisphosphonate-related osteonecrosis of the jaw (BRONJ), a painful condition in which bone cells in the jaw bone die, often leading to infection, exposed bone, and the need for extensive oral surgery. While it is said to be a rare complication of bisphosphonates, thirty patients with BRONJ were written up by Israeli researchers recently.[9] In some patients, the BRONJ extended into nearby structures like the nose and the sinuses.

Many of these patients had cancer. Bisphosphonates are also used to prevent further bone loss in people who have multiple myeloma, a malignancy that affects the bone marrow, or in people with other forms of cancer that have spread, or metastasized, to the bone. And while most of the people in the article were receiving bisphosphonates in the setting of malignancies, some did not have cancer and were being treated for osteoporosis. The estimated incidence of BRONJ in people treated with intravenous bisphosphonates is up to 12.8 percent in people with multiple myeloma and up to 12 percent in women with metastatic breast cancer.

There is no completely effective treatment for BRONJ, so when it occurs in people with osteoporosis, they may be condemned to suffer this side effect for many years, unlike people with malignancies who may have a very limited life expectancy. These same authors reported on eleven women without cancer who developed BRONJ after taking oral bisphosphonates for osteoporosis.[10] They pointed out that Merck, the manufacturer of the most widely prescribed oral bisphosphonate, alendronate, estimates that the incidence of this complication is only 0.7 per one hundred thousand person years. But in Israel, about one hundred thousand people a year are prescribed oral bisphosphonates, and the authors estimate that twenty to twenty-five patients in the country suffer from this complication. They therefore believe that Merck is underestimating the risk of bisphosphonate-related osteonecrosis of the jaw.

Another serious side effect that has recently come to light with the use of the intravenous bisphosphonate Reclast, is kidney damage. From April 2007 until February 17, 2009, the FDA's Adverse Event Reporting System (AERS) received reports of twenty-four cases of kidney impairment and acute kidney failure associated with the use of Reclast.[11] The FDA concluded, "Although some cases noted underlying medical conditions and/or concomitant medications, there were cases in which it was possible to establish a reasonable association between Reclast and the event."

The Cautionary Tale of DES Use in Pregnant Women

Probably the most egregious example of an FDA-approved drug that had severe, unintended side effects was diethylstilbestrol, also called DES. This medicine, a synthetic estrogen, was prescribed between 1950 and 1970 to women to prevent miscarriage, despite the fact that there was little evidence that it was effective in this regard. In 1971 an article in the *New England Journal of Medicine* noted the association of a rare type of tumor of the vagina, clear cell adenocarcinoma (CCA), in young women who had been exposed to DES in utero—that is, their mothers had taken the drug while pregnant with them.[12] These tumors were diagnosed at a median age of nineteen, with a range of fifteen to twenty-two. No one knows exactly how many women were exposed to DES in utero, but it is thought to be in the millions. Estimates of the rate of development of CCA in DES-exposed women range from one in one thousand to one in ten thousand.[13] Once this association became known, women who had been exposed to DES in the womb had to undergo multiple examinations and repeated biopsies so that early diagnosis might allow them to be saved.

Not only was there a heightened risk of this rare cancer, but both women and men exposed to DES before birth had a higher incidence of congenital abnormalities. These included small, abnormally shaped wombs, and abnormalities of the Fallopian tubes that often led to miscarriages. In the sons of women who had taken DES while pregnant, there was an increased risk of abnormalities in the development of the testes and penis. As the authors noted at the end of this article: "Ultimately, the DES story humbles us. It serves as a reminder that though the narrow lens of today might reassure us that an intervention is safe, it is only with the wisdom of time that the full consequences of our actions are revealed."

The distortion of medical research by Big Pharma is pervasive. As Dr. Angell noted in her *Boston Review* article, "Industry-supported research is far more likely to be favorable to the sponsors' products than is NIH-supported research." Negative results may never be published. If a clinical trial does not yield a finding that is favorable for the drug being studied, the report may never see the light of day. In a Pfizer-sponsored study called CASHMERE (Carotid Atorvastatin Study in Hyperlipidemic Postmenopausal Women), 192 women beyond menopause were randomized to 80 milligrams daily of atorvastatin (Lipitor), while 206 women were randomized to placebo. They had a measurement called carotid intima-media thickness (CIMT) ascertained by an ultrasound examination of the carotid artery at the beginning of the study and twelve months later to see if there was less of an increase in CIMT in the women on atorvastatin, compared to the women on placebo. Less of an increase in CIMT would have been a positive result, a sign that the statin had slowed progression of atherosclerosis.

But, in fact, women on atorvastatin had a slightly *greater* increase in CIMT than did the women on placebo. If the opposite had occurred, you can be certain this would have been touted as yet another reason to treat women with atorvastatin. Not surprisingly, the results of the CASHMERE study were never published in a medical journal. You can find them after a lot of digging at Clinical Study Results Database (www.clinicalstudyresults.org.), a website launched by the trade association Pharmaceutical Research and Manufacturers of America (PhRMA).

Illegal Activity on the Part of Big Pharma

Over the last decade, more and more evidence of illegal pharmaceutical company activity has come to light, in some cases because of information supplied by whistle-blowers. Between January 2001 and September 2009, eighteen federal fraud cases against Big Pharma were settled, with fines of $8,672,000. Some of these involved off-label marketing (promoting drugs for nonapproved uses); others concerned submitting inaccurate price data to the government, paying kickbacks to induce prescribing, or offering rebates to private insurers.[14]

Industry Influence on Professional Medical Associations (PMAs)

Industry influence is also rife in PMAs like the American College of Cardiology (ACC), the American College of Physicians (ACP), and the American Heart Association (AHA), to name but a few. The PMAs bring together physicians with common specialties and interests, sponsor continuing medical education (CME) opportunities, hold annual meetings at which new research findings are presented, write guidelines for practitioners, lobby Congress, publish prestigious medical journals, and define ethical norms for their members. Any real or perceived conflict of interest, therefore, has the potential for great harm.

As a 2009 article in the *Journal of the American Medical Association* reported regarding PMAs, "Industry funding of their activities, although varying in degrees, is pervasive." Funding takes many forms. Big Pharma and medical device companies often purchase booths in the exhibit halls found in the convention centers where scientific meetings are held. In these booths, they distribute gifts and pamphlets describing their products. In addition, these same companies often give physician attendees grants for travel to the meetings, sponsor lavish free dinners, and hold other social events.[15]

Industry also supports the medical journals put out by PMAs by buying advertising space, and industry funds underwrite many accredited continuing medical education courses offered by the PMAs, while also supporting the publication and dissemination of practice guidelines. Furthermore, pharmaceutical companies support medical journals by ordering thousands of copies of articles reporting on favorable clinical trials, which their sales reps then hand out to physicians during sales visits to doctors' offices.

Does Industry Money Influence the AHA?

The amounts of money involved are staggering. Take the American Heart Association (AHA), for example. The AHA is a nonprofit organization with a mission to "build healthier lives free of cardiovascular disease and stroke." It actively solicits donations from individuals and companies, and reports assets of almost $1 billion.[16]

Integrity in Science (ISS), a project of the organization Center for Science in the Public Interest (CSPI), reviews studies and other scientific literature for conflicts of interest between researchers and industry. As detailed on its website, "For the fiscal years from 03–04 to 06–07, AHA reports receiving $30,158,173 from pharmaceutical and medical device companies."[17] Thirty million dollars can buy a lot of influence.

Contributions from industry help to support lavish salaries for AHA executives. In 2008 the AHA paid CEO M. Cass Wheeler a whopping $1,089,331 in salary and an additional $53,238 from the AHA and "related organizations"—for a thirty-eight-hour workweek.[18] This is many multiples of what your average primary care doctor earns working sixty hours a week. With this kind of money at stake, the AHA is unlikely to espouse positions that would compromise Big Pharma profits.

The AHA also rakes in millions of dollars each year from other corporate sources: namely, food companies, which pay big bucks to gain the "heart-check mark" imprimatur from the AHA. The foods so anointed have to be low in fat, saturated fat, and cholesterol. The Integrity in Science website notes that the AHA charges anywhere from $5,490 to $7,500 per product in the first year to give permission to add the heart-check mark to a product's label. There are hefty renewal fees each year.

What are some of these supposedly heart-healthy foods? Would you believe a whole list of processed meats, including Boar's Head All Natural Ham (340 milligrams of sodium in a 2-ounce serving) and Boar's Head EverRoast Oven Roasted Chicken Breast (440 milligrams of sodium in a 2-ounce serving)? In order to be classified as "low sodium," according to FDA guidelines, a food has to contain 140 milligrams of sodium or less, but apparently the AHA is not interested in the salt content of the food it endorses. This, despite the fact that a high sodium intake raises blood pressure, thus increasing the risk of ASCVD. And you have to wonder if these meats are from animals who were pumped full of hormones and antibiotics to accelerate their growth and maximize profits for the large conglomerates that have taken over most food production in the United States.

Not only is processed meat high in sodium, but there is excellent evidence that eating even just one serving a day increases the risk of diabetes as well as heart disease. In a review of almost 1,600 studies that included more than one million people in ten countries on four continents, the authors of a recent meta-analysis showed that a 1.8-ounce daily serving of processed meat raised the risk of diabetes by 19 percent and of heart disease by 42 percent.[19] The list of supposedly heart-healthy foods also includes lots of "reduced" fat or "lean" ground beef. But the leanest ground beef still contains 4 percent saturated fat, which is way too much, especially given the supersized portions many people consume.

But drugs, medical devices, and foods are not the only potential sources of income that the American Heart Association has tapped. In May 2010 the AHA was taken to task in the media for endorsing Nintendo's Wii gaming system. As reported by MedPage Today in an article entitled "Is Wii Worthy of an AHA Endorsement?," Nintendo paid the AHA $1.5 million over three years for an "exclusive relationship."[20] In an interview, Dr. Clyde Yancy, president of the AHA, defended the endorsement, despite doubts about the amount of exercise that Wii users will actually achieve. The article quotes Janet Fulton, an epidemiologist at the US Centers for Disease Control and Prevention (CDC): "The amount of activity one achieves from this active gaming is really inconclusive in terms of its benefit on health."

In the same article, Dr. Yancy was asked about another product that carries the AHA heart-check mark: a drink called Chocolate Moose Attack. The interviewer pointed out that this beverage contains more sugar per ounce than regular Pepsi. Dr. Yancy defended the AHA's decision by saying that "the totality of the product is what we have to evaluate. Low fat, low sodium. We have to look at the entirety of the package."

How can the AHA's recommendations about diet, not to mention drugs, be trusted when the organization is so beholden to Big Pharma and giant food corporations? Simply put, they can't be. These recommendations were bought and paid for, and we consumers are the losers.

Reining in Big Pharma

So what can be done to rein in the influence of Big Pharma on the medical profession and professional medical associations? In order to help avoid conflicts of interest, the authors of the *JAMA* article on PMAs and their relationship to industry made recommendations based on five premises.

First, that pharmaceutical and medical device companies *do* make important contributions to medical practice and that "resolving issues of conflicts of interest is not best accomplished by avoiding all relationships."

Second, the premise underlying the recommendations is the unequivocal demonstration by various research studies that gifts to physicians *do* have the power to influence physicians' choices.

Third, education must be distinguished from marketing.

Fourth, ties to industry take various forms, so guidelines must take all of these into account.

Fifth, PMAs must set their own agendas, and "proposed industry support for a project should not alter the agendas of PMAs."

Some of the concrete recommendations in the article were that PMAs should work toward a total ban on pharmaceutical and medical device industry funding, except for that derived from journal advertising and exhibit hall fees. At the annual meeting of the American College of Cardiology, literally acres of space are taken up by booths sponsored by Big Pharma, medical device companies, makers of stress-testing equipment, and so on, hawking their wares and giving away goodies (the most popular of which seems to be espresso, with thumb drives coming in a close second).

The authors of the *JAMA* article admit that the goal of zero percent financing is unrealistic in the short term, and suggest that PMAs adopt an interim goal of having no more than 25 percent of their operating budgets supplied by industry sources. They also recommend that PMAs should avoid taking part in industry marketing activities and stipulate that PMA leaders, as well as the members of the committees that write the all-important practice guidelines, should be free of any conflicts of interest.

Most pertinent to this book is that last recommendation. Practice guidelines influence how doctors diagnose and treat people, and set "evidence-based" standards for decision making in medical practice. As noted in chapter 1, the National Cholesterol Education

Program and its Expert Panel on Detection, Evaluation, and Treatment of High Blood Cholesterol in Adults has published guidelines for LDL cholesterol goals based on whether or not someone is considered at "low risk" (LDL cholesterol goal is less than 160), "intermediate risk" (LDL cholesterol goal is less than 130) and "high risk" or "established vascular disease or its equivalent" (LDL cholesterol goal is less than 100). These guidelines recommend drug therapy when therapeutic lifestyle changes are insufficient to get people to a certain level of LDL cholesterol.

When the guidelines were updated in 2004 to recommend an "optional LDL cholesterol goal" of less than 70 in people with vascular disease and multiple risk factors—a level that is usually impossible to achieve without high doses of statins—few people knew that eight of the nine scientists promulgating this recommendation had financial ties to pharmaceutical companies that manufacture cholesterol-lowering drugs. Is it not naive to think that they were totally unswayed by their Big Pharma paymasters?

A study of just how rife conflicts of interest are among the scientists who establish clinical practice guidelines (CPG) was published in the Archives of Internal Medicine in 2011.[21] These guidelines make recommendations for the treatment or prevention of various cardiac conditions, including ASCVD, heart failure, heart attacks, and abnormal heart rhythms. The authors of this paper examined the seventeen most recent practice guidelines from the American College of Cardiology and the American Heart Association, and found that more than 56 percent of the 498 individuals writing the guidelines reported conflicts of interest. Commenting in the same issue of the Archives, Dr. Steve Nissen of the Cleveland Clinic wrote, "No conceivable logic can defend the practice of including promotional speakers and stockholders on CPG writing committees."[22] Indeed.

In April 2010 the Council for Medical Specialty Societies (CMSS) proposed a new Code for Interactions with Companies to "improve integrity and transparency."[23] The code addresses research funding, company sponsorship, donations, and industry influence on medical meetings, clinical practice guidelines, journals, licensing, and advertising. It is a twenty-eight-page document that broadcasts its naiveté in the preamble, when it admits that although Big Pharma and medical device companies are for-profit entities, they "also strive to help patients live longer and healthier lives. Companies invest resources to bring new drugs, devices, and therapies out of the laboratory and to the patient while maximizing value for shareholders."

Only the gullible would believe that maximizing value for shareholders comes in second to helping patients in Big Pharma's scheme of things.

Key principles of the code for medical societies include independence (PMAs will foster independence from industry in the development of educational activities and scientific programs) and transparency (PMAs will make their policies regarding conflicts of interest known to both their members and the general public). There are suggestions covering the acceptance of corporate sponsorship, educational grants for society meetings, and CME events, and so forth and so on. But the code has no teeth.

The code is purely voluntary and has been described as "weak" and "vague" to the point of being "almost humorous" in a communication from theheart.org, a website for cardiologists and other health care professionals, on May 4, 2010.[24] The impetus for the code was a series of investigations by Iowa senator Charles Grassley's office into payments to physicians, and concerns about the influence of industry on medical practice raised by the Institute of Medicine. There's nothing like a snooping legislator to stir some housekeeping efforts on the part of medicine and Big Pharma.

The American College of Cardiology (ACC) signed on to the code and updated it so that it is more stringent than the CMSS code. The ACC now requires that 50 percent of the guideline and performance-measure writing groups, plus the chairperson, can have "no relevant ties to industry." Apparently it's okay for the other 50 percent to be bought and paid for by Big Pharma. Dr. Steven Nissen of the Cleveland Clinic called the CMSS code "lacking in courage" and went on to say, "This document is really a smokescreen . . . There's nothing in here that prevents professional societies from accepting large amounts of money from industry."

———

As this chapter has made clear, much current medical research is tainted by both real and potential conflicts of interest. With billions of dollars in sales at stake, Big Pharma suppresses negative results and exaggerates positive results in clinical trials of the drugs it manufactures. Prominent academic medical centers, professional medical associations, and physicians have huge financial incentives to expand the indications for treatment—a glaring example of which is the use of statins in healthy patients with normal levels of cholesterol, based on the flawed JUPITER trial. For millions of people to spend billions of dollars on drugs that have serious side effects, for minimal benefit, makes no sense, particularly when there are lifestyle modifications that can be extremely beneficial, with no risk of side effects. It makes sense only if you are Big Pharma or someone who holds the patent on, say, a blood test of questionable value.

Never has it been more important to be an informed consumer.

Fearmongering and Selling Sickness

Before we close this look at Big Pharma, one further disturbing trend needs to be mentioned. In a telling article, "Selling Sickness: The Pharmaceutical Industry and Disease Mongering," which appeared in the *British Medical Journal* (*BMJ*) in 2002,[25] the authors wrote, "There's a lot of money to be made from telling healthy people they're sick. Some forms of medicalising ordinary life may now be better described as disease mongering."

Baldness, shyness, restless legs, difficulty sleeping, heartburn, difficulty obtaining an erection—all relatively common human conditions or experiences—are turned into diseases with frightening-sounding names: alopecia, social phobia, restless leg syndrome, insomnia, gastroesophageal reflux disease, erectile dysfunction. And—surprise, surprise—all can be treated with expensive medicines that will "cure" these new "diseases." Direct-to-consumer marketing of drugs for these and many other conditions influence people to think that there is a pill out there somewhere that will treat anything that bothers them. It is impossible to watch television for thirty minutes without seeing advertisements for medicines to treat these dubious conditions. Patients then pressure their physicians to prescribe medicines they see advertised on TV. Valuable resources that could be put to better use elsewhere are squandered.

And Americans are still no healthier. The rates of obesity and diabetes soar as we continue our sedentary ways and eat food that is calorically dense but nutritionally poor. In the immortal words of the cartoon character Pogo, "We have met the enemy and he is us." Presented with huge portions of relatively inexpensive processed foods, we succumb to inadvertent gluttony. Empowered by ever more sophisticated machines, we fall victim to facilitated sloth. And we wonder why our waistlines continue to expand.

I hope that the foregoing chapters have persuaded you that a prescription for statins should not be taken lightly. Chances are that your physician does not know that even if you've already had a heart attack, you can lower your risk of another without lowering your LDL cholesterol, as was shown in the Lyon Diet Heart Study.

I hope that if you do suffer muscle pain from statins but the blood tests show "no muscle damage," you can educate your doctor about the evidence that statin-induced muscle damage can occur without the blood test being abnormal.

And I hope that you will be willing to question your physician if she or he wants you to take a statin. To re-cap, you need to ask the questions that are listed at the end of chapter 1 before you start a statin medication.

The following chapters will provide you with more detailed information about the heart, the scientific method, clinical research, and healthy eating.

Part 3

A CLOSER
LOOK AT THE
SCIENCE

Chapter 8

The Heart and Its Discontents: What Happens in Sickness and in Health

Some of the information in this chapter was touched on briefly in chapter 1, but here I will go into greater detail about this critical organ. To understand the importance of your heart, you need to know what it does. Basically, your heart is a muscular pump. Its job is to pump blood throughout the body so that your cells can obtain the oxygen and nutrients they need to survive and perform their myriad functions. After blood has picked up fresh oxygen in the lungs, the arteries carry it away from the left side of the heart. Arteries divide into smaller and smaller branches until they become microscopic vessels with very thin walls, called *capillaries.* These capillaries (in all organs except the lungs) deliver oxygen and nutrients to the cells, and take in carbon dioxide and other waste products of metabolism. (*Metabolism* refers to the series of chemical reactions that takes place within our cells so that they can grow, maintain the integrity of their cell walls, reproduce themselves, and interact with other cells.)

Veins are blood vessels that carry the blood that has been depleted of oxygen and nutrients back to the right side of the heart. This venous blood then gets pumped into the lungs where carbon dioxide is given up and oxygen is taken in. The pulmonary veins carry this blood into the left atrium, then the newly enriched blood is ready to be pumped out by the left side of the heart, and the cycle of circulation begins again.

The human heart has four chambers: two receiving chambers, the *right atrium* and the *left atrium* (*atrium* is a Latin word referring to the entrance room in ancient Roman villas); and two pumping chambers, the *right ventricle* and the *left ventricle*. The artery that routes blood to the lungs is called the *pulmonary artery*, and the artery that distributes blood to the rest of the body is called the *aorta*. Four one-way valves keep the blood traveling through the heart in the correct direction. On the right side of the heart, the valve between the right atrium and the right ventricle is called the *tricuspid valve*, and the valve between the right ventricle and the pulmonary artery is called the *pulmonic valve*. On the left side of the heart, the valve between the left atrium and the left ventricle is called the *mitral valve*, and the valve between the left ventricle and the aorta is called the *aortic valve*. Figure 1, a schematic drawing of the heart, shows its interior structure.

At times these heart valves can malfunction. Sometimes they become narrowed, or *stenotic*, and sometimes they leak. A mildly narrowed or leaky valve is not a cause for concern. These valvular malfunctions are best diagnosed by a simple, safe test called an

Figure 1: The Heart

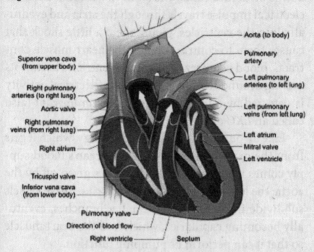

Superior vena cava (from upper body)

Right pulmonary arteries (to right lung)

Aortic valve

Right pulmonary veins (from right lung)

Right atrium

Tricuspid valve

Inferior vena cava (from lower body)

Pulmonary valve

Direction of blood flow

Right ventricle

Aorta (to body)

Pulmonary artery

Left pulmonary arteries (to left lung)

Left pulmonary veins (from left lung)

Left atrium

Mitral valve

Left ventricle

Septum

With permission from the National Heart, Lung, and Blood Institute, National Institutes of Health, US Department of Human Services, www.nhlbi.nih.gov/health/dci/Diseases/hhw/hhw_anatomy.html.

echocardiogram, or *cardiac ultrasound.* This test uses sound waves to construct pictures of the beating heart.

Sometimes patients come to me very frightened because their primary care doctor has told them, based on such a test, that they have a leaky valve. I tell them that it's a bit like gray hair and wrinkles. If you live long enough, your hair turns gray, your skin wrinkles, and your valves start to leak. If valves become very narrowed or very leaky, that is more serious but, nowadays, fixable.

The heart also has an electrical system. Electrical impulses normally start high in the right atrium in a little structure called the *sinus node*. From here the electrical impulse travels through the atria and eventually into the ventricles, giving them a little shock that causes them to contract. When the heart muscle contracts, blood is squeezed out of the ventricles to start its cycling around the body. The heart's electrical activity is detected by a test called an *electrocardiogram* (also called an *EKG* or an *ECG*).

Like all pumps, the heart needs energy, which it gets from the oxygen in the blood. The organ's blood supply comes from the first two branches given off by the aorta: the left and right coronary arteries. These vessels subdivide into smaller and smaller branches, eventually becoming capillaries, which feed the heart muscle so that it can perform its pumping function.

Normally the heart contracts, or beats, about sixty to one hundred times per minute—depending on your age and activity level—as it pumps blood around the body. That means that over an average life span of eighty years, the heart contracts and relaxes an astounding three billion times. That's pretty impressive, by any criteria. If your heart is damaged to the extent that it can't pump enough blood to meet the body's needs, a condition called *congestive heart failure* ensues. People with this condition are short of breath with activity, and may even be breathless at rest if their heart failure is severe. If your heart stops beating for more than four or five minutes, you suffer irreversible brain damage and die. Since the health of the heart is integral to the health of the whole body, it's pretty obvious why it is so important to safeguard your heart.

Many diseases can affect the heart, but the most common one is atherosclerosis. The word was first introduced in 1904 by Felix Marchand, a German pathologist, who suggested that atherosclerosis was the process most often responsible for obstructing arteries. The word is derived from two Greek words: *athera,* meaning "porridge" or "gruel"; and *scleros,* meaning "hard." The pathologists who first examined arteries containing what we now call plaque thought that it looked like porridge and noted that it had a hard consistency.

One of the earliest signs of atherosclerosis is called the "fatty streak." These lesions are made up of specialized white blood cells that have eaten up (phagocytized) cholesterol. In the developed world, the process of atherosclerosis begins in childhood. In fact, researchers have reported finding fatty streaks in the aortas of spontaneously aborted fetuses from mothers who had high levels of cholesterol in their blood.[1]

We are still unraveling what happens as plaque builds up in arteries; for reasons that are not totally understood, veins do not build up plaque. We do know that anything that injures the artery, such as smoking, makes it more apt to develop plaque.

Arteries are made up of three layers. The thin, innermost layer, called the *intima,* or *endothelium,* forms the main protective barrier against harmful agents that may travel in the blood, such as carbon monoxide and other poisons given off by cigarette smoke. The next layer, the *media,* is made up mainly of smooth muscle cells that can contract and relax, allowing the artery to constrict in response to something like hemorrhage or to dilate in response to anything that increases the demand for blood, such as exercise. The outermost layer is called the *adventitia,* and it is made up mainly of *connective tissue,* which gives support to the artery. The opening of the artery through which blood flows is called the *lumen.*

Multiple agents can injure the innermost wall of the artery, among them high levels of LDL cholesterol, high blood pressure, high levels of blood sugar as is seen in diabetes, and many of the toxins in cigarette smoke. When LDL cholesterol enters the blood vessel wall, it sets off an *inflammatory reaction* (from the Latin word *inflammare,* meaning "to set on fire"). Inflammation is the body's attempt to seal off an area of injury, remove it, and begin the process of healing the damage. Key to the inflammatory process is a special kind of white blood cell called a *monocyte.* When monocytes sense inflammation, they rush to the site and turn themselves into *macrophages* (literally "big eaters," from the Greek words *macros* for "large" and *phagein* for "eat"), which gobble up the LDL cholesterol particles and, in the process, become what are called *foam cells.* Over time, with recurrent injury to the vessel wall, these foam cells accumulate, smooth muscle cells and fibrous tissue cells migrate into the intima in an attempt to wall off the injury, and the resultant plaque can start to narrow the arterial lumen, obstructing the blood flow. The plaque becomes covered by a *fibrous cap,* a covering of scar tissue that walls off the plaque and its contents from the bloodstream.

Figure 2 is a schematic drawing of a normal artery and an artery that has plaque buildup.

Figure 2: An Artery with Plaque Buildup

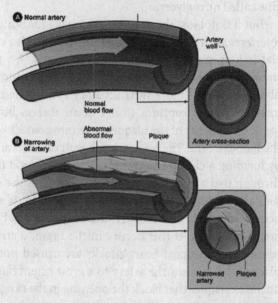

With permission from the National Heart, Lung, and Blood Institute, National Institutes of Health, US Department of Human Services, www.nhlbi.nih.gov/health/dci/Diseases/Cad/CAD_WhatIs.html.

If a coronary artery develops so much plaque that not enough blood reaches the heart muscle, *ischemia* results. Heart muscle that is starved for oxygen is said to be *ischemic*, and people who have ischemic heart muscle often experience the symptom we call angina pectoris (from the Latin words *angina*, meaning "strangling or choking," and *pectoris,* meaning "of the chest"). The hallmark of angina is that it is predictably brought on by exercise or emotional stress and goes away in a few minutes with rest, relaxation, or a medicine called nitroglycerin.

But it is not just the extent to which plaque buildup interferes with blood flow that is important. Also crucial is how stable or unstable the plaque is. An unstable plaque is one with more liquid fat, a thinner fibrous cap, and more inflammatory cells. When an unstable plaque ruptures (think of an abscess bursting), the contents of the plaque come into contact with the bloodstream. The body tries to wall off this injury by forming a clot. If the clot totally blocks blood flow through that artery, the tissue downstream of the clot dies unless blood flow is restored promptly. If this occurs in the heart, a heart attack (myocardial infarction) results. If this occurs in the brain, a stroke results. In fact, most heart attacks are caused not by plaques that narrow the artery to a great extent but by unstable plaques that block the opening in the range of 10 percent to 40 percent.

―――――

During the first half of the twentieth century, cardiovascular disease increased steadily. In the United States, heart disease became the leading cause of death in 1921, and stroke took the number three position in 1938. However, going back to 1950—long before the era of bypass surgery, statins, stents, and other miracles of modern medicine—the age-adjusted death rate (which takes into account the differences in age distribution across a population) from cardiovascular disease began to decline. In the more than sixty years since then, it has fallen by some 60 percent.[2]

The epidemic of CVD began to garner the attention of investigators in the aftermath of World War II when, perhaps not coincidentally, millions of young GIs became nicotine addicts, compliments of the tobacco companies that saw it as their patriotic duty to supply them with free cigarettes included in C rations.[3]

The Framingham Heart Study is the best known of the investigations that established the risk factors for CVD. A risk factor is anything that increases one's risk of developing a disease. It can be a behavior (like being a couch potato or smoking), an abnormal accumulation of something in the blood (such as glucose or cholesterol), a treatable condition (like high blood pressure), or something unavoidable (such as age or a genetic defect). This information, discussed in chapter 1, bears repeating.

The study, which began in 1948, recruited two-thirds of the inhabitants of Framingham, Massachusetts, between the ages of thirty and sixty-two, to participate in a long-term trial intended to pinpoint the risk factors for developing CVD. The volunteers agreed to come in every other year for blood samples, examinations, and to fill out questionnaires about their health status. As a result of the Framingham Heart Study and many other investigations, we learned that there are only two risk factors for CVD that are not modifiable: age (forty-five and above for men, fifty-five and above for women) and family history. Every other risk factor is modifiable, avoidable, or treatable. They include smoking, sedentary lifestyle, obesity, abnormal levels of cholesterol and other blood fats, diabetes, high blood pressure, and inflammation.

Atherosclerotic cardiovascular disease is quintessentially a lifestyle disease. But as we've grown addicted to calorically dense, nutritionally deficient fast food, overweight if not obese (two-thirds of Americans), and far too often too busy or too lazy to exercise, we prefer to believe that a pill will take care of the damage we inflict on our bodies.

Big Pharma is complicit in this charade. The drug companies make money by selling drugs; they make nothing (in fact, they stand to lose money) if people eat heart-healthy, plant-based diets, stop smoking, lose weight, and exercise. And so, with an eye always on the bottom line, Big Pharma got into the business of clinical research. In chapter 9, I'll go into greater detail about the studies that were used to justify treating people with cholesterol-lowering medicines.

Chapter 9

Clinical Research and the "Science" Being Used to Support Statin Use

Before we take a closer look at clinical trials, a brief explanation of the scientific method is in order. We human beings are driven to make sense of the world around us. We have a particular interest in discerning the causes of phenomena and in predicting the future. For thousands of years, occurrences like volcanic eruptions, floods, and plagues were attributed to gods, malign spirits, or witches, and the like. Ancient Romans tried to predict the future by examining the entrails of animals or observing the flights of birds. We may scoff at them for what we now consider superstition, but ancient Romans were extremely talented engineers, not to mention conquerors of much of the then known world. And while some ancient sages, like Aristotle and the medieval Islamic scholar-physician Avicenna, made early attempts at what we would classify as a "scientific method," it wasn't until the Renaissance of the fourteenth through seventeenth centuries that significant changes occurred in the way we viewed the world and the methods by which we sought to explain natural phenomena.

During the Renaissance, a process for discovery—a scientific method—was honed and applied in various disciplines. Francis Bacon, the English philosopher and scientist, was one of the first to lay out its principles. In astronomy, the method led to the discoveries of Copernicus and Galileo. In medicine, it led to the accurate depictions of human anatomy by Andreas Vesalius and the discovery of the circulation of the blood by the English physician William Harvey. Indeed, every field of knowledge benefited from the application of the scientific method.

This new way of thinking relied heavily on *empiricism*: the theory of knowledge that emphasizes the role of experience and evidence. Rather than relying on intuition, religious dogma, or revelation, the scientific method postulates that truth can be arrived at by formulating hypotheses and testing them in controlled experiments. (Merriam-Webster's dictionary defines *hypothesis* as "a tentative assumption made in order to draw out and test its logical or empirical consequences.") Needless to say, many Renaissance practitioners of the scientific method were feared and persecuted by religious authorities. Going up against religious dogma in those days could get you tortured on the rack or burned at the stake.

In its modern form, the scientific method has four steps:

1. Observe and describe a phenomenon.
2. Formulate a hypothesis to explain the phenomenon.
3. Make predictions based on the hypothesis.
4. Design and perform experiments to prove or disprove the hypothesis.

One might add, especially in the era of Big Pharma, a fifth step: publicize the results of these experiments.

The application of the scientific method helps to prevent errors from creeping into our thinking. It helps to separate *association* (a grouping of phenomena or entities) from *causation* (the act of causing something to happen). As an example of the types of errors that can arise by confusing association with causation, think of two graphs, one illustrating the sales of sneakers in the United States since 1970, and the other illustrating the rates of obesity in the United States since 1970. Both graphs would show steady increases, but to say that increased use of sneakers *caused* the increased rates of obesity would be absurd. Unfortunately, in the realm of medical research, conflating association with causation has all too often led us down the wrong path.

With regard to the epidemic of cardiovascular disease that took place in the twentieth century, scientists observed that people with high levels of cholesterol in the blood were more likely to develop atherosclerotic cardiovascular disease (ASCVD). This led to the so-called cholesterol hypothesis that cholesterol causes ASCVD. (See chapter 2.) This was a gross oversimplification of a complex issue. As we learned earlier, it is the levels of various lipoproteins that are important (that is, high levels of VLDL cholesterol and LDL cholesterol, and low levels of HDL cholesterol), not simply the total cholesterol level.

But getting back to the scientific method, once scientists had hypothesized that high levels of LDL cholesterol "caused" ASCVD, the only way that they could prove or disprove this hypothesis was to devise experiments to test the hypothesis. The mechanism for doing so became known as the clinical trial. These studies allow us to determine if an intervention (be it a drug, an operation, a device, and so on) is beneficial or not. They also allow us to prove or disprove a hypothesis—in this case, that lowering elevated levels of LDL cholesterol lowers the risk of ASCVD.

Clinical trials are different from observational studies, in which individuals—for example, postmenopausal women taking hormone replacement therapy (HRT)—are observed over time, and various outcomes (for example, the number of heart attacks or bone fractures) are measured. Observational studies are not experiments. No attempt is made to intervene with a drug or other therapy. And they are subject to what is called *selection bias*. For example, postmenopausal women who decide to take hormone replacement medicines might be less likely to be obese and to smoke. These factors could undermine and skew a comparison with women in the general population. In order for observational studies to be valid, the people selected for such a study must be similar to one another and to the rest of the population. Otherwise the conclusions drawn from the study may not be valid.

As it turns out, many observational studies noted that women who took hormone replacement therapy—estrogen and progesterone—after menopause had a lower incidence of heart disease than women who did not take HRT. But when HRT was studied in a randomized, placebo-controlled, double-blind trial (the Women's Health Initiative Postmenopausal Hormone Therapy trial), no benefit of HRT was found. In fact, women on hormone replacement therapy suffered more heart attacks and strokes than the women who took a placebo. A likely explanation of these different findings is that the women who chose to take HRT in observational studies (since this wasn't under the control of the investigators) were healthier and had fewer risk factors than women who didn't take HRT; they therefore had a lower risk of ASCVD that had nothing to do with HRT. Again, association should not be confused with causation.

Application of the scientific method has spurred the huge increase in knowledge that the human race has accumulated over the last few centuries. It has brought us vaccines; life-saving drugs, devices, and operations; computers; the Internet; and trains, planes, and automobiles. But it has also brought us weapons of mass destruction. With that sobering thought in mind, let us now take a closer look at how the story of cholesterol

and heart disease evolved over the last decades of the
twentieth century.

Early Clinical Trials in Heart Disease

The first clinical trial that sought to prove that lowering cholesterol lowered the risk of coronary heart
disease events was the Coronary Drug Project.[1] This
study, begun in 1966, recruited 8,341 men between
the ages of thirty and sixty-four who had survived
a heart attack (therefore it was a secondary prevention trial), and randomized them to five treatment
regimens or a placebo. Statins had not been invented
yet, and we didn't have very good drugs to lower cholesterol. Doctors knew that among the drugs that
exerted this effect were the female hormone estrogen (Premarin), thyroid hormone, large doses of the
B vitamin niacin, and clofibrate (Atromid-S), a medicine of the fibrate class. (Fibrates mainly lower triglyceride levels, and if you lower those, you usually
also lower cholesterol).

The participants were treated with one of these
medicines or a placebo and followed prospectively
(that is, over a period of time) to see how they fared.
There were actually two estrogen doses, a high dose (5
milligrams per day) and a low dose (2.5 milligrams per
day). After an average follow-up of only one and a half
years, the high-dose estrogen group was told to stop the
study drug because more men in this group were having heart attacks and dying compared to the placebo
group. In 1973, after an average follow-up of 4.7 years,

the low-dose estrogen group was told to stop the study drug. The reasons were twofold: not only was there no benefit compared to placebo, but the men were complaining bitterly of a side effect called *gynecomastia*, or breast enlargement. Thyroid hormone and clofibrate treatment did not demonstrate any benefit, but after an average of six years of treatment with niacin, there was a modest benefit in reducing nonfatal heart attacks in this one treatment arm compared to placebo, which persisted after fifteen years.[2]

In the midseventies, two other clinical trials sought to demonstrate the impact of lowering cholesterol on the occurrence of cardiac events. The Program on the Surgical Control of the Hyperlipidemias (POSCH) trial used a surgical approach to lowering cholesterol, so it was not exactly a blinded trial. (You can't fake a surgical scar.) The surgery, a partial ileal bypass, shortens a portion of the small intestine in order to increase the excretion of bile acids from the body and to lower levels of LDL cholesterol (more on that below). The Lipid Research Clinics Coronary Primary Prevention Trial (LRC-CPPT) used a bile acid sequestrant drug called cholestyramine (Questran), which lowers cholesterol in the blood by binding to bile acids and increasing their excretion from the body. This was a randomized, double-blind, placebo-controlled study.

Our bodies produce about 800 milligrams of cholesterol a day, about half of which is oxidized to form bile acids, which are important in the digestion of fats and in removing cholesterol from the body. Bile acids are stored in the gallbladder. After a fatty meal, the gallbladder contracts to push the bile acids into the small intestine. There they emulsify fats, making them absorbable. Most of these bile acids get reabsorbed in the last part of the small intestine, called the terminal ileum. This process is called the *enterohepatic circulation*. If you interrupt this enterohepatic circulation of bile acids, the body tries to compensate by converting more cholesterol to bile acids, and thus the level of cholesterol in the blood drops. The POSCH trial interrupted the enterohepatic circulation by surgically bypassing the terminal ileum.

Between 1975 and 1983, 838 survivors of a documented heart attack who had high cholesterol levels were recruited into the POSCH study: 417 were assigned to dietary treatment to lower cholesterol (control group) and 421 to diet plus partial ileal bypass surgery (intervention group).[3] They were then followed prospectively to determine the number in each group who died from any cause, or from coronary heart disease (CHD). The study was unusual for its era because it included some women, albeit only 78, or 9.3 percent of the total group.

The formal POSCH trial ended on July 19, 1990, after an average follow-up of 9.7 years. Partial ileal bypass led to a 23.3 percent greater reduction in total plasma cholesterol and a 37.7 percent greater reduction in LDL cholesterol at five years in the intervention group compared with the control group. Overall deaths and deaths due to CHD were decreased in the surgical group compared to the control group, but this result was not statistically significant.

However, the surgically treated group in the POSCH trial did have a relative risk reduction of 35 percent if you combined two end points: nonfatal heart attacks and deaths due to CHD. Out of 417 people in the control group, 125 had either a nonfatal heart attack or CHD death (30 percent), compared to 82 out of 421 people (19 percent) in the surgical group. (The relative risk reduction is calculated by subtracting the rate of cardiac events in the experimental group from the event rate in the control group, divided by the event rate in the control group.)

But if you look at absolute risk reduction, the results don't seem so impressive, because the absolute risk reduction is the difference between 30 percent and 19 percent—or 11 percent. When researchers present the results of clinical trials, and particularly when Big Pharma publicizes the results of successful trials, they report the relative risk reduction because it always sounds more impressive than the absolute risk reduction, which may be quite small even though it is statistically significant.

The Lipid Research Clinics (LRC) trial was the first primary prevention trial of a cholesterol-lowering drug: cholestyramine.[4] This study recruited 3,806 middle-aged men who had high levels of LDL cholesterol but did not have symptoms or a diagnosis of heart disease. It was the early 1970s, and at the time I was a young doctor at the National Heart, Lung, and Blood Institute, working in the program office that designed the trial and oversaw the many centers around North America where the study was conducted. This experience kicked off my interest in treating patients with high cholesterol and in preventing ASCVD.

The men were randomized to either the active drug or a placebo; both groups were put on a moderate cholesterol-lowering diet. Diet alone reduced LDL cholesterol by 5 percent to 6 percent in both groups. The group that received cholestyramine saw its LDL cholesterol drop by an additional 26 percent, while those in the placebo group had a 5 percent reduction in LDL cholesterol.

After an average of 7.4 years of follow-up, the men who got cholestyramine experienced a 19 percent relative risk reduction in the primary end point, which was death definitely due to CHD and/or nonfatal heart attack. This result was statistically significant—that is, the p value was less than 0.05. But again, the absolute risk reduction was rather puny, with a primary end point occurring in 8.6 percent of the men on placebo compared to 7 percent of the men on cholestyramine: an absolute risk reduction of only 1.6 percent.

As mentioned before, this happens again and again when clinical trial results are reported. The relative risk reduction (in heart attacks or whatever is defined as the primary end point) is the number that is always published because it sounds more impressive than the absolute risk reduction, which may be on the order of only a few percentage points. On the other hand, when reporting *adverse effects* of drugs, the absolute risk of people having a side effect is reported, not their risk relative to people not taking the drug. Researchers and

Big Pharma do this because the latter number would be more alarming.

Once statins were approved by the FDA, there was a great impetus to study just how effective they were in both primary prevention of ASCVD (preventing the clinical manifestations of disease in people who have no signs or symptoms) and secondary prevention (preventing further events in people who already had ASCVD). I've already discussed some of these trials in chapters 2 and 4, but now I'll go into them in greater detail.

Starting in the 1990s, many large trials using statin drugs were undertaken. Most compared a statin to placebo, but some compared statin to "usual care," or low-dose statin to high-dose statin. Some just looked at the hard end points of nonfatal heart attack and cardiac death. Others used composite end points that were softer, like "the need for revascularization." This "need" was often determined by the person's physician, not the physicians carrying out the study, and there is wide variability in the alacrity with which physicians decide whether or not to refer a patient for revascularization. In the final analysis though, what we should be most focused on is whether or not treatment lowers one's risk of dying from any cause. For example, a drug might lower the risk of dying from heart disease, while at the same time increasing the risk of dying from cancer, in which case the risk of dying from any cause might be unchanged.

So what happens if we look at all-cause mortality in people treated with statins?

Let's consider primary prevention first. In an article published in 2010, the authors analyzed the results of eleven primary prevention trials that compared statins to placebo and looked at all-cause mortality.[5] Despite the fact that the participants in these trials did not have established cardiovascular disease, they were all considered to be at high risk of ASCVD because of various risk factors. For example, some of the trials included people with diabetes. The studies went by catchy names such as JUPITER, ALLHAT, ASCOT, MEGA, AFCAPS/TexCAPS, WOSCOPS, PROSPER, CARDS, ASPEN, PREVEND IT, and HYRIM. The results of the individual trials were reported between 1995 and 2008. The total number of participants was 65,229, and the average age was between fifty-one (PREVEND IT) and seventy-five (PROSPER), with an overall average age of sixty-two years. Not surprisingly, there was a significant relationship between age and mortality rates, with the highest mortality rate occurring in the study with the highest average age.

Sixty-five percent of the participants were men and 35 percent were women. (The range of female participation in these trials varied from 0 percent to 68 percent.) The average follow-up was 3.7 years. The mortality rates were given as the number of deaths per one thousand person years—in other words, the number of deaths per one thousand people over one year. The mortality rate was 11.4 per one thousand person years in people on placebo and 10.7 per one thousand person years in people on statins. This was not a statistically significant difference. In other words, chances are that the small difference noted was due to chance. There was also no relationship between the amount that LDL cholesterol was reduced and all-cause mortality. The authors concluded: "This literature-based meta-analysis did not find evidence for the benefit of statin therapy on all-cause mortality in a high-risk primary prevention set-up."

What about secondary prevention with statins? There is no meta-analysis comparable to the one mentioned above for primary prevention, but if we consider three large secondary prevention trials of statins, we find that in people with established vascular disease, treatment with statins did reduce overall mortality. The first of these studies to be reported was the 4S trial, which stands for the Scandinavian Simvastatin Survival Study.[6] In a neat coincidence, this study randomized 4,444 participants with established vascular disease to either simvastatin (Zocor) or placebo. Over a median follow-up of 5.4 years, 12 percent of people in the placebo group died compared to 8 percent of people in the statin group, and this was a statistically significant difference.

The next secondary prevention trial I've included was the LIPID (Long-Term Intervention with Pravastatin in Ischaemic Disease) study.[7] This trial included 9,014 people with established coronary artery disease and randomized them to either pravastatin (Pravachol) or placebo. During an average follow-up of 6.1 years, overall mortality was 14.1 percent in the placebo group and 11 percent in the statin treated group. This was also a statistically significant difference.

The last and largest of these secondary prevention trials was called HPS, or the Heart Protection Study.[8] This trial followed 20,536 people for an average of five years. The total mortality rate was 14.7 percent in people taking placebo and 12.9 percent in people taking simvastatin—a significant difference.

Among the 33,994 participants in these three trials (4S, LIPID, and HPS) the all-cause mortality was decreased by 4 percent, 3.1 percent, and 1.8 percent, respectively. So even though statins do not decrease the risk of dying when given to people without vascular disease, they do lower the risk of dying in people with vascular disease, albeit by only a few percentage points. But remember, diet alone, in the Lyon Diet Heart Study, also decreased the risk of dying.

In chapter 10, I'll provide you with delicious, easy-to-prepare recipes that incorporate the foods associated with the Mediterranean diet. Eating these foods is guaranteed *not* to make your muscles ache, *not* to damage your brain and nerves, and *not* to increase your risk of diabetes.

Part 4

THE SAFE, DELICIOUS STATIN ALTERNATIVE

Heart-Healthy Foods
and Recipes, and Two Weeks of
Mediterranean Diet Menus

My interest in healthy eating dates back to childhood. My parents were influenced by one of the first people to advocate for unprocessed food, nutritionist-author Adelle Davis. Among her best-selling books was *Let's Have Healthy Children*, first published in 1951, and since my parents were raising ten of us, they wanted to be sure that their food budget dollars were being spent wisely. White sugar and white bread were banned from our table. Our lunch boxes contained whole wheat sandwiches (which meant that our friends wouldn't trade their sandwiches for ours, much to our dismay), and we put brown sugar on our oatmeal at breakfast, or no sugar at all.

My mother drank a concoction called "Tiger's Milk," which she mixed from skim milk, brewer's yeast, black-strap molasses, and wheat germ. It was a distinctly unappetizing brown color and had an indescribable taste I can still remember, but she remained healthy (and, perhaps more surprisingly, sane) while giving birth to ten children in ten years. Another interesting fact was that her cholesterol was over 300 every time it was measured. She never took a statin, did not have heart disease, and lived to be eighty-eight before succumbing to complications of hydrocephalus (also known as "water on the brain," hydrocephalus is an abnormal collection of brain fluid). Needless to say, her HDL cholesterol—the good kind—was quite high.

My introduction to the Mediterranean diet occurred in childhood also, although we did not call it that in those days. My father used to sell life insurance in an Italian neighborhood in the Bronx, New York. Some of his customers were very hospitable and pressed homemade food on him. He fell in love with Italian cooking and bought an Italian cookbook. He brought it home to my mother and said, "Here, learn how to cook like this." So she did, and I grew up eating pizza, pasta, olive oil, and classic dishes like eggplant parmigiana and chicken cacciatore.

My experiences as a practicing physician cemented my belief in the importance of a healthy diet. I give a copy of the menus in this chapter to every patient in my practice and ask them about their diet at every visit. These are dishes that we eat at home, since I don't believe in asking my patients to do something that I'm unwilling to do myself. The menus at the end of the chapter incorporate the recipes given below. So, read, enjoy, and as my Italian-American in-laws say, "Mangia, mangia!" Eat, eat!

Eating for Heart Health

Most of us try to eat three meals a day, so I'll start by providing lists of heart-healthy foods for breakfast, lunch, dinner, and snacks. These will be followed by recipes incorporating the principles of the Mediterranean diet. Lastly, I will provide two weeks of menus for breakfast, lunch, and dinner.

HEART-HEALTHY BREAKFAST FOODS

Oatmeal

Hard-boiled eggs with olive oil

Yogurt and fruit

Whole wheat toast

Eggs fried in olive oil

Heart-healthy muffins (see recipes)

Omelets

HEART-HEALTHY LUNCH FOODS

Tuna fish salad

Spinach salad with hard-boiled eggs

Mixed green salad with chickpeas

Vegetarian whole wheat pizza

Egg salad

Sardine, onion, and red lettuce sandwich on whole wheat bread

Smoked salmon and cream cheese on whole wheat bagel

HEART-HEALTHY DINNER FOODS

Fish, especially oily fish such as salmon

Any vegetable, the more colorful the better

Legumes (beans)

Hearty vegetarian soups served with crusty bread

Shellfish, including shrimp, lobster, and clams

Risottos (rice dishes)

Whole wheat pasta with vegetable or seafood
topping

HEART-HEALTHY SNACKS

Unsalted nuts

Dried fruit

Heart-healthy muffins (see recipes)

Dark chocolate

Fresh fruit

Heart-healthy cookies (see recipes)

Heart-healthy cakes (see recipes)

RECIPES

Northern Beans

Ingredients

  2 15.5-oz cans cannellini or northern beans or
      2 cups dried beans
  1 shallot
  1 medium red onion
  1 cup extra-virgin olive oil (or more to taste)
  6 cloves garlic, chopped
  2 tsp dried oregano
  2 tsp dried basil
  1 tsp dried thyme
  ½ tsp dried red pepper flakes (or more to taste)
  1 bay leaf
  Salt and pepper to taste
  1 14.5-oz can of diced tomatoes
  1 cup white wine
  Crusty Italian bread, preferably whole wheat
  Fresh flat-leaf parsley, chopped (optional)
  Freshly grated parmesan cheese

Soak two cups of dried cannellini or northern beans
overnight, rinse, then boil until tender in salted water. If using cans of precooked beans, rinse well and
drain.

In a Cuisinart or food chopper, chop the shallot and onion into small pieces. In a saute pan, cook
the chopped shallot and chopped onion in half of the
extra-virgin olive oil until they are translucent, about
5 to 7 minutes. Add the garlic, spices, salt, pepper, diced

tomatoes, and white wine. Simmer for 10 minutes. Add the beans and simmer for an additional 30 minutes, stirring frequently.

Toast a piece of crusty Italian bread and drizzle with extra-virgin olive oil. Top with the beans and more olive oil, some chopped flat-leaf parsley if you have it, and freshly grated parmesan cheese. These beans are even better the second day, as they've had more time to absorb the flavors.

Serves four to six.

Wasabi-Roasted Salmon

Ingredients

- ¼ cup to ½ cup Inglehoffer Hot Creamy Wasabi
  (depending on amount of salmon)
- ¼ cup to ½ cup mayonnaise
- 1 salmon fillet, between ¾ pound and 1 pound

Combine equal amounts of the Inglehoffer Hot Creamy
Wasabi and the mayonnaise. Mix well. Spread over top
(non-skin side) of salmon fillet. Bake skin-side down in
a preheated 450-degree oven for about 19 minutes for a
thick fillet and 17 minutes for a thin fillet.

Serves three to four.

Cioppino

Ingredients

- ¾ cup extra-virgin olive oil
- 1 medium onion, chopped
- 5 cloves garlic, minced
- 2 celery stalks, chopped
- ½ cup white wine
- 1 tbsp lemon juice
- 3 tbsp fresh flat-leaf parsley, chopped
- Salt and pepper to taste
- 1 28-oz can Italian crushed tomatoes
- 2 bay leaves
- 3 fillets of cod or snapper
- 2 lobster tails, cut up
- 12 shrimp, shelled and deveined
- 12 scallops
- Clams, mussels, oysters, crab legs, if desired
- Crusty Italian bread, preferably whole wheat

Saute the first eight ingredients in a large pot for about 5 to 10 minutes over medium heat. Add the tomatoes and bay leaves and cook for 30 minutes over medium heat. Add cod or snapper. Cook on low for about 20 minutes.

In a separate pot, boil the lobster and remaining seafood until just done. Don't overcook. Stir in the tomato mixture and serve with crusty Italian bread.

Serves six to eight.

Cod Provençale

Ingredients

    4 cod fillets, about 6 oz to 8 oz each
    1 large red or yellow onion, diced
    6 cloves garlic, chopped
    2 14.5-oz cans diced tomatoes
    3 stalks celery, diced
    ½ cup extra-virgin olive oil
    4 tbsp capers
    12 chopped Kalamata olives (pits removed)
    1 tsp dried oregano
    1 tsp dried basil
    ¼ tsp black pepper
    Salt to taste

Preheat oven to 450 degrees. Saute onion and garlic in the olive oil over medium heat for 5 minutes. Add the tomatoes, celery, capers, olives, herbs, pepper, and salt. Simmer over low heat for about 10 minutes. Arrange the cod fillets in a 9 x 13–inch baking dish. Spoon the tomato mixture over the fillets. Bake in a preheated oven for 10 to 15 minutes.

Serves four.

Shrimp Remoulade

My brother Edwin Hudson who manages Raoul's restaurant in Manhattan made this dish for us while we vacationed in Maine over the summer. The recipe came from Raoul's immensely talented chef David Honeysett, who was happy to share it.

Ingredients

- 4 to 5 lbs medium to large shrimp
- 3 oz Dijon mustard
- 6 oz mayonnaise
- 9 oz shrimp cocktail sauce
- 1 bunch scallions, thinly sliced
- 6 interior celery stalks
- ¾-bunch fresh flat-leaf parsley, chopped
- Kosher salt and black pepper to taste

Boil the shrimp for 4 to 8 minutes depending on the size. Allow to cool, then peel and devein. Dice the celery. Mix together the mustard, mayonnaise, cocktail sauce, salt, and pepper. Add the thinly sliced scallions, diced celery, chopped parsley, and shrimp. Fold together, then chill in the refrigerator for at least 4 hours before serving. May be served as an appetizer, or over lettuce as a salad.

Marinara Sauce

Ingredients

>   1 large red or yellow onion, diced
>   6 large cloves garlic, finely chopped
>   1 28-oz can Italian plum tomatoes
>   6 anchovy fillets in oil
>   1 cup extra-virgin olive oil
>   ½ cup dry white wine
>   ¼ tsp dried red pepper flakes
>   Salt and black pepper to taste

Place olive oil in large saucepan over medium heat. Mash up the anchovy fillets and add to the oil. Add the onions and cook until they are translucent, about 5 to 10 minutes. Add the garlic and cook an additional 5 minutes. Add the tomatoes, white wine, and seasonings. Continue to cook over low heat, stirring frequently, until the liquid has cooked down and you have a thick sauce.

Porcini Mushroom Sauce

Ingredients

- 1 oz dried porcini mushrooms
- 1½ cups warm water
- 1 large yellow onion, diced
- ½ cup no-trans-fat margarine
- ½ cup olive oil
- 1 28-oz can Italian plum tomatoes
- Salt and black pepper to taste

Rinse dried mushrooms and place in a bowl of warm water. Allow to rehydrate for at least 1 hour, then drain, reserving all the water, which will have turned a deep brown. Chop the mushrooms into approximately ½-inch pieces. Saute the onion in the margarine and olive oil until translucent. Add the mushrooms, reserved liquid, and tomatoes. Season with salt and pepper to taste. Cook over low heat, stirring frequently, until you have a thick sauce.

Pasta with Avocado Sauce

Ingredients

> 2 ripe avocados
> ½ cup to 1 cup extra-virgin olive oil
> ½ cup capers
> 2 cloves garlic, thinly sliced
> Salt and black pepper to taste
> ½ lb fettuccine, preferably whole wheat
> Freshly grated parmesan cheese

Peel a very ripe avocado and cut into bite-sized cubes. Peel another avocado and mash with ½ cup of extra-virgin olive oil. (You may need more, depending on the size of the avocado; you should be able to pour the mixture.) Drain capers. Add capers and garlic to the mashed avocado–olive oil mixture. Cook whole wheat fettuccine according to directions on package. Drain well and pour the avocado-caper-garlic-oil mixture over the warm pasta, adding more olive oil if necessary. Add the cubed avocado and toss lightly. Top with freshly grated parmesan cheese and serve immediately.

Serves two to three.

Pasta Puttanesca

I've read various explanations as to why the name of this dish translates as "whore's pasta," or "harlot's pasta." In Nancy Verde Barr's We Called It Macaroni, *she writes that it was so named because the ladies of the night were able to cook it up quickly between clients. I've also read that in the old days, harlots were allowed to shop only one day a week, so their ingredients needed to be able to keep well in establishments that might not boast ice-boxes or refrigerators. In any event, this dish is a great favorite with my family.*

Ingredients

5 anchovy fillets

1 large red onion, diced

6 cloves garlic, finely chopped

1 28-oz can Italian crushed tomatoes

¾ cup extra-virgin olive oil

½ cup red wine

¼ cup capers

1 cup brine-cured black olives, such as Kalamatas

1 tbsp dried oregano

1 tbsp dried basil

¼ cup fresh flat-leaf parsley, chopped

Freshly grated parmesan cheese

1 lb dried pasta, preferably whole wheat

Mash the anchovy fillets and saute in olive oil with the onion on low heat, about 5 minutes or until the onion is translucent. Add the garlic and cook for an additional 4 to 5 minutes. Add the rest of the ingredients, except the cheese and pasta, and cook over low heat, uncovered, until some of the liquid has evaporated and the sauce has thickened. Stir frequently. This will take about 20 to 30 minutes.

Boil about 5 quarts of water and add the dried pasta. Cook according to directions. (Cooking time will depend on what shape and size of pasta you choose.) Drain pasta in a colander and toss with the sauce. Top with freshly grated parmesan cheese.

Serves four to six.

Farfalle and Beans

Ingredients

2 15.5-oz cans small white beans
1 cup extra-virgin olive oil
1 medium red onion, diced
4 cloves garlic, finely minced
½ cup fresh flat leaf parsley, chopped
12 sun-dried tomato halves (in oil)
Zest and juice of 2 lemons
Salt, black pepper, and celery salt to taste
½ lb farfalle (also called bow-tie) pasta, preferably whole wheat

Put beans in a colander, rinse well, and allow them to drain. Place in a large serving bowl and add the olive oil, onion, and garlic. Julienne the sun-dried tomato pieces and add them to the bowl, along with the lemon zest, lemon juice, and seasonings. Mix well.

Bring 4 quarts of water to a boil and add the pasta. Cook according to instructions on the package until the pasta is semifirm, or al dente. Remove from heat, drain the pasta, and rinse with cool water. After the pasta is well drained, add to the bean mixture and stir well. Serve cold or at room temperature.

Serves four to six.

Shrimp Kebabs

Ingredients (to make 4 kebabs)

> 16 jumbo shrimp, peeled and deveined
>
> 4 ripe tomatoes, quartered
>
> 4 medium red onions, quartered
>
> 4 sweet bell peppers (red, orange, and yellow),
>   seeded and quartered
>
> 1 20-oz can pineapple chunks
>
> ½ cup to 1 cup extra-virgin olive oil
>
> Salt, black pepper, and garlic powder
>
> 4 metal or wooden skewers

If using wooden skewers, soak them in water for at least 30 minutes. Alternately thread the skewers with the shrimp, tomatoes, onions, peppers, and pineapple, using 4 shrimp per skewer. Mix the olive oil with seasonings. Brush over the kebabs.

Preheat a broiler or an outdoor grill. If using a grill, spray with nonstick spray. Grill the kebabs, turning once and basting with olive oil until the shrimp is just cooked through, about 4 to 5 minutes.

Serves two to four.

Sauteed Flounder

Ingredients

   4 skinless flounder fillets, 4 oz to 6 oz each
   1 egg
   All-purpose flour for dredging
   Salt and black pepper to taste
   Bread crumbs
   Fresh flat-leaf parsley

Beat the egg with a fork until it's a uniform color. Dredge the flounder in flour that has been seasoned with salt and pepper. Coat the flounder with beaten egg, then dredge in bread crumbs. Saute in olive oil about 3 to 4 minutes per side, until browned. Garnish with fresh parsley and serve with lemon wedges.

Serves four.

Sole Piccata

Ingredients

> 4 sole fillets, 4 oz to 6 oz each
> All-purpose flour for dredging
> Salt and black pepper to taste
> 4 tbsp olive oil
> 4 tbsp no-trans-fat margarine
> ½ cup white wine
> Zest and juice of one lemon
> 2 tbsp drained capers
> ½ cup fresh flat-leaf parsley, chopped

Dredge the sole fillets in flour seasoned with salt and pepper. Heat a large frying pan over medium-high heat, then add the olive oil and half the margarine. When the oil bubbles, add the fish fillets and cook over high heat, turning once, until they are well browned, about 2 to 3 minutes per side. Remove fish to a warmed platter and add wine to the pan, scraping up any browned bits. Add lemon zest and juice and capers and continue to cook down for about a minute, and then add the last 2 tablespoons of margarine. Return the fish to the pan to rewarm. Garnish with parsley and serve.

Serves four.

Angie's Cabbage

My mother-in-law, Angelina Avarista, made this dish for Sunday dinner many years ago, and I've been serving it in our home ever since.

Ingredients

    1 medium-sized head green cabbage
    ¾ cup extra-virgin olive oil (or more to taste)
    Salt and black pepper to taste
    6 to 10 large cloves garlic, finely chopped
    ½ cup dry white wine (optional)
    1 14.5-oz can diced tomatoes

Cut cabbage head into quarters, then julienne into ¼-inch slices. Add the olive oil to a large skillet and place over high heat. Add the shredded cabbage and cook, stirring frequently, allowing cabbage to brown but not burn. Add salt and pepper to taste. After all the cabbage is wilted, add the garlic, white wine, and tomatoes. Continue cooking until most of the liquid is cooked off.

Serves six to eight.

Escarole and Bean Soup

This soup hits the spot on a wintry New England day.

Ingredients

1 head (bunch) of escarole
1 cup extra-virgin olive oil (or more to taste)
4 large shallots, diced, or 1 large red onion, diced
6 to 10 cloves garlic, chopped
1 tbsp dried oregano
1 tbsp dried basil
1 tbsp dried parsley
¼ tsp dried red pepper flakes (or more to taste)
Salt and black pepper to taste
2 15.5-oz cans great northern beans, drained and rinsed
½ cup dry white wine (optional)
8 cups vegetable broth
Freshly grated parmesan cheese

Cut off the bottom of the escarole head, rinse well, drain, and chop the escarole leaves. Set aside. In a large skillet, heat the olive oil and add shallots or onion. Saute, stirring frequently, until translucent, about 5 minutes. Add garlic and cook for an additional 5 minutes. Add escarole, oregano, basil, parsley, red pepper flakes, salt, and pepper. Cook for an additional 5 to 10 minutes until escarole leaves are wilted. Mash 1 can of the beans into a paste and add, along with the other can of whole beans, wine, and vegetable broth to the escarole-herbs mixture. Bring to a boil and cook for an additional 10 to 15 minutes. Ladle into soup bowls, and just before serving, grate parmesan cheese over the top.

Serves six to eight.

Lemon-Pineapple Muffins

Ingredients

- 1 whole lemon
- 6 slices canned pineapple (drain and reserve the liquid)
- ¾ cup brown sugar
- ½ cup plus 2 tbsp Smart Balance or other no-trans-fat margarine
- 1¼ cups all-purpose flour
- ¼ cup wheat germ
- ¾ cup dried cranberries (may substitute raisins or chopped dried dates)
- ¾ cup chopped walnuts
- 1 tsp kosher salt
- 1 tsp baking powder
- 1 tsp baking soda
- 1 large egg
- ½ cup reserved pineapple liquid

Preheat oven to 400 degrees. Mix all the dry ingredients in a large mixing bowl. Wash the lemon and cut the unpeeled lemon in half lengthwise, then slice each half into several ¼-inch pieces, removing the seeds but conserving as much of the juice as possible. (Cut and deseed the lemon over a large bowl to save the juice.) Add lemon pieces, and saved juice, pineapple slices, and margarine to a Cuisinart or blender and mix until well pureed. Add to dry ingredients, along with the egg and pineapple liquid. Mix dry and wet ingredients until just blended; don't overmix. Spoon into greased muffin pans and bake for approximately 20 to 25 minutes or until the tops are golden brown.

Makes about 15 to 18 muffins.

(These muffins freeze well in a ziplock bag or other airtight container. To defrost, just pop a muffin in the microwave on high for 30 seconds.)

Zucchini Walnut Bread

Ingredients

   2½ cups all-purpose flour
   ½ cup wheat germ
   1 tsp salt
   1 tsp baking powder
   1 tsp baking soda
   3 tsp ground cinnamon
   3 eggs
   1 cup canola oil
   1 tsp vanilla extract
   2 cups light brown sugar
   2 cups zucchini, grated
   1 cup walnuts, coarsely chopped

Grease two 8 x 4–inch loaf pans. Preheat oven to 350 degrees. Mix flour, wheat germ, salt, baking powder, baking soda, and cinnamon in a bowl. In a separate large bowl, mix the eggs, oil, vanilla, and brown sugar until well blended. Add to the dry ingredients and beat well. Add grated zucchini and walnuts and stir until well mixed. Pour batter into greased pans. Bake for 50 to 60 minutes or until a toothpick inserted in the center comes out clean. Cool for 20 minutes, then remove from pans and allow to cool completely. If you want to freeze, cover completely in plastic wrap, place in a zip-lock bag, and store in the freezer.

Cocoa-Carrot Muffins

Ingredients

    4 cups baby carrots
    8 slices canned or fresh pineapple
    1½ cups brown sugar
    1¼ cups Smart Balance or other no-trans-fat margarine
    2½ cups all-purpose flour
    ½ cups wheat germ
    ½ cup unsweetened cocoa
    1½ cups dried cranberries
    1½ cups walnuts, chopped
    2 tsp salt
    2 tsp baking powder
    2 tsp baking soda
    2 eggs
    1 cup pineapple juice

Preheat oven to 400 degrees and grease muffin pans. Cream together sugar, margarine, and cocoa. Grate carrots and puree pineapple slices. Add them along with the eggs to the creamed sugar mixture along with pineapple juice and mix well. Add nuts and cranberries and mix well. Add dry ingredients and mix until just blended. Drop batter into muffin pans and bake at 400 degrees for 15 to 17 minutes. Makes about three dozen. Allow to cool completely. May be frozen in air-tight containers.

Orange Muffins

Ingredients

- 1 whole seedless orange
- ½ cup plus 2 tbsp no-trans-fat margarine
- ¾ cup brown sugar
- 1 egg
- ½ cup orange juice
- 1 tsp kosher salt
- 1 tsp baking soda
- 1 tsp baking powder
- 1¼ cups all-purpose flour
- ¼ cup wheat germ
- ¾ cup dried cranberries (may substitute raisins or chopped dried dates)
- ¾ cup walnuts, chopped

Preheat oven to 400 degrees. Combine dry ingredients in a large mixing bowl. In a Cuisinart or blender, puree the whole unpeeled orange, after cutting into about 8 pieces, with the margarine. Add to the dry ingredients along with the egg and orange juice. Mix until just blended; do not over mix. Spoon into greased muffin tins and bake for about 20 minutes. This recipe makes about 18 muffins. They can be frozen in ziplock bags after they cool completely.

Almond Butter Cookies

Almonds are higher in protein than any other nuts. They are also rich in monounsaturated fat, which raises the level of HDL (good) cholesterol. They are a great source of vitamin E, folic acid, fiber, and calcium. These cookies are a huge hit with children of all ages.

Ingredients

    1½ cups brown sugar
    ¾ cup no-trans-fat margarine
    2 eggs
    16 oz almond butter (1 jar)
    2 tbsp truffle honey (may substitute plain honey)
    ½ tsp almond extract
    ½ tsp vanilla extract
    1½ cups all-purpose flour
    ½ cup wheat germ
    2 cups quick oats oatmeal
    2 tsp baking soda
    1 tsp cinnamon
    ½ tsp nutmeg
    1 cup walnuts, coarsely chopped
    1 cup dried cranberries (may substitute raisins or
        chopped dried dates)

Preheat oven to 350 degrees. (If using a convection oven, preheat to 325.) Combine sugar and margarine until well blended. Add eggs one at a time. Add almond butter, honey, almond and vanilla extracts, and beat until smooth. In a separate bowl, combine dry ingredients. Add to wet ingredients and stir until just incorporated. Stir in walnuts and cranberries. Drop by a generous rounded tablespoonful 1½ inches apart on greased baking sheets. Bake for 12 to 15 minutes until golden brown on top. Let cool completely, then remove to cookie plate.

The recipe makes 4 to 5 dozen cookies. These cookies may be frozen in air-tight containers after they have cooled completely.

Macadamia Nut Cookies

These cookies combine the goodness of macadamia nuts and dark chocolate. Macadamia nut oil has the highest percentage of monounsaturated fat of any food. These nuts are also high in fiber and the B vitamin thiamine. Dark chocolate is rich in flavonoids, phytochemicals that combat inflammation. Studies have also shown that dark chocolate can relax blood vessels and help prevent strokes and blood clots. Most of all, these cookies are just plain delicious.

Ingredients

¾ cup plus 2 tbsp all-purpose flour

¼ cup wheat germ

½ tsp baking soda

¼ tsp salt

½ cup no-trans-fat margarine

½ cup brown sugar

1 large egg

1 tsp vanilla extract

9 oz Ghirardelli Intense Dark chocolate bar, coarsely chopped

1 cup dry-roasted, nonsalted macadamia nuts, coarsely chopped

Preheat oven to 375 degrees. In a mixing bowl, cream together the margarine and sugar. Add the egg and vanilla extract. Combine dry ingredients and add to mixing bowl. Add the chocolate and macadamia nuts. Drop by heaping tablespoonsful onto greased cookie sheets 2 inches apart. Bake for 12 to 15 minutes or until golden brown.

Makes about 2 dozen cookies.

Carrot Bundt Cake

Carrots are free of saturated fat, high in fiber, and a great source of vitamin A. That might explain why it can be hard to get your family to eat them. But if you jazz them up with canola oil, dried cranberries, walnuts, brown sugar, and spices, I guarantee that your family and guests will change their opinions of the humble carrot.

Ingredients

  1½ cups all-purpose flour
  ½ cup wheat germ
  4 eggs
  1¼ cups canola oil
  1½ cups brown sugar
  2 tsp vanilla extract
  2 tsp baking powder
  2 tsp baking soda
  ½ tsp kosher salt
  2 tsp ground cinnamon
  ½ tsp ground nutmeg
  4 cups baby carrots, grated
  1 cup dried cranberries
  1 cup walnuts or pecans, chopped
  Rum or brandy for marinade
  confectioners sugar

Marinate the dried cranberries in rum or brandy for at least 2 hours. Just before making the cake, drain them and set aside. Preheat oven to 350 degrees. Grease and lightly flour a large Bundt pan. In a large mixing bowl, beat together eggs, oil, sugar, and vanilla extract. Mix in dry ingredients. Add carrots, marinated cranberries, and nuts. Pour into a prepared pan and bake until toothpick inserted in cake comes out clean, about 50 to 60 minutes. Let cool in pan for 10 minutes, upend over serving plate, and remove Bundt pan when completely cooled. Dust with confectioners sugar.

Two Weeks of Mediterranean Diet Menus

While some of these meals would seem foreign to people living in the countries bordering the Mediterranean Sea, they all incorporate the basic tenets of the Mediterranean diet: that is, they are plant based; they feature colorful fruits and vegetables, whole grains, legumes (beans), and seafood; and they use olive oil as the main source of fat calories. I have left out usual breakfast accompaniments such as coffee, tea, and juice, but add them if you wish.

WEEK ONE ———————————————

Monday

Breakfast: Oatmeal topped with fresh or thawed frozen berries and nuts (walnuts, almonds, or pecans).

Lunch: Tossed salad made with baby spinach, canned beet slices, black and green olives, sun-dried tomatoes in oil, sunflower seeds, chickpeas, or other beans, and dressed with extra-virgin olive oil and red wine or balsamic vinegar.

Dinner: Pasta with avocado sauce and mixed green salad. Fresh or dried fruit for dessert and a glass of wine (if your doctor allows).

Tuesday

Breakfast: Lemon-pineapple muffins.

Lunch: Tuna fish salad sandwich with lettuce and tomato on whole wheat bread.

Dinner: Salmon with creamy wasabi topping, roasted sweet potatoes, and spinach sautéed in olive oil. Carrot Bundt cake for dessert and a glass of wine (if your doctor allows).

Wednesday

Breakfast: Whole wheat pancakes topped with fruit, nuts, and honey.

Lunch: Northern beans.

Dinner: Shrimp kebabs with brown rice and broccoli sautéed in olive oil. Fresh or dried fruit for dessert and a glass of wine (if your doctor allows).

Thursday

Breakfast: Hard-boiled eggs topped with olive oil or eggs scrambled in olive oil; whole wheat toast.

Lunch: Farfalle and beans.

Dinner: Pasta puttanesca with salad of baby spinach, kiwi fruit, and walnuts topped with extra-virgin olive oil and rice wine vinegar. Fresh or dried fruit for dessert and a glass of wine (if your doctor allows).

Friday

Breakfast: Whole wheat toast spread with organic almond butter and honey.

Lunch: Caprese salad (fresh tomatoes, buffalo mozzarella, and fresh basil drizzled with extra-virgin olive oil and balsamic vinegar).

Dinner: Sauteed flounder fillets with roasted fingerling potatoes and acorn squash. Almond butter cookies for dessert and a glass of wine (if your doctor allows).

Saturday

Breakfast: 4 oz of 1 percent yogurt (preferably Greek) topped with fruit and nuts.

Lunch: Almond butter and jelly sandwich on whole wheat bread.

Dinner: Sole piccata with roasted sweet potatoes and broccoli rabe sauteed in olive oil and garlic. Fresh or dried fruit for dessert and a glass of wine (if your doctor allows).

Sunday

Breakfast: French toast (preferably made with whole wheat bread) topped with fresh or frozen strawberries and chopped walnuts.

Lunch: Tofu burger on whole wheat bun or bread with lettuce and tomato.

Dinner: Cioppino served with crusty Italian bread and mixed green salad. Fresh or dried fruit for dessert and a glass of wine (if your doctor allows).

WEEK TWO

Monday

Breakfast: Omelet made with onions and sun-dried tomatoes.

Lunch: Sardine, onion, and red lettuce sandwich on rye bread.

Dinner: Broiled salmon with boiled red potatoes and sauteed broccoli. Fresh or dried fruit for dessert and a glass of wine (if your doctor allows).

Tuesday

Breakfast: Zucchini walnut bread.

Lunch: Escarole and bean soup.

Dinner: Pasta with porcini mushroom sauce and a mixed green salad. Macadamia nut cookies for dessert and a glass of wine (if your doctor allows).

Wednesday

Breakfast: Orange muffins.

Lunch: Almond butter with sliced bananas and honey sandwich on whole wheat bread.

Dinner: Whole wheat pasta with marinara sauce and a mixed green salad. Fresh or dried fruit for dessert and a glass of wine (if your doctor allows).

Thursday

Breakfast: Eggs scrambled in olive oil with whole wheat toast.

Lunch: Smoked salmon and cream cheese on whole wheat bagel.

Dinner: Broiled tuna steak with roasted sweet potatoes and sauteed broccoli rabe. Fresh or dried fruit for dessert and a glass of wine (if your doctor allows).

Friday

Breakfast: Cocoa carrot muffins.

Lunch: Northern beans with crusty Italian bread.

Dinner: Cod provençale with roasted red potatoes and Angie's Cabbage. Almond butter cookies for dessert and a glass of wine (if your doctor allows).

Saturday

Breakfast: Omelet made with onions, mushrooms, and grated parmesan cheese.

Lunch: Swiss cheese, tomato, and lettuce sandwich on whole wheat bread.

Dinner: Baked sea bass with couscous and acorn squash. Fresh or dried fruit for dessert and a glass of wine (if your doctor allows).

Sunday

Breakfast: Zucchini omelet with whole wheat toast.

Lunch: Crab meat salad with sliced avocado and tomato.

Dinner: Boiled lobster with mashed red potatoes and sauteed spinach. Carrot Bundt cake for dessert and a glass of wine (if your doctor allows).

GLOSSARY

Abdominal obesity (also called **visceral obesity**): defined as a waist measurement of more than forty inches in men and more than thirty-five inches in women. It is one of the components of the metabolic syndrome.

Amyotrophic lateral sclerosis (ALS): a degenerative disease affecting the nervous system that leads to muscle wasting, weakness, and eventual death. Also called Lou Gehrig's disease.

Angina (also called **angina pectoris**): a symptom caused by insufficient blood flow to the heart muscle. It is usually experienced as a squeezing, burning, or pressure discomfort in the chest that is brought on by exercise or emotional upset and goes away within a few minutes with rest, relaxation, or a medicine called nitroglycerin.

Angiogram: a diagnostic procedure in which dye is injected into a blood vessel and X-ray pictures are taken.

Angioplasty: a procedure that is performed on narrowed arteries to increase the size of the blood vessel's opening. It involves advancing a special balloon-tipped catheter across the narrowing, then inflating the balloon to widen the artery.

Antioxidant: a substance that inhibits the process of oxidation.

Aorta: the main artery that leaves the left side of the heart.

Aortic valve: the valve between the main pumping chamber on the left side of the heart, the left ventricle, and the aorta.

Arteriosclerosis: hardening of the arteries.

Artery: a blood vessel that carries oxygenated blood to our organs (except the pulmonary artery, which carries unoxygenated blood from the heart to the lungs).

Atherosclerosis: a specific form of hardening of the arteries in which a complex substance called plaque builds up in the arteries.

Atherosclerotic cardiovascular disease (ASCVD): a disease caused by the buildup of plaque in the arteries supplying the heart and/or other organs.

Atorvastatin (trade name, **Lipitor**): a statin medication used to treat high levels of LDL cholesterol.

Atrium (plural, **atria**): the upper, receiving chambers in the heart.

Autonomic nervous system (ANS; also called the **visceral nervous system**): the part of the nervous system that supplies nerves to our internal organs, blood vessels, and the glands that manufacture hormones.

Body mass index (BMI): a measurement calculated by dividing one's weight in kilograms by one's height in meters, multiplied by itself. Normal values are between 18.5 and 24.9.

Capillaries: the smallest blood vessels, visible only through a microscope. From the capillaries (except in the lung), oxygen and nutrients are delivered to cells. In the lung capillaries, carbon dioxide is given up, and oxygen is taken in by the blood.

Carbohydrates: one of the major food classes. Too much of this food class in the diet leads to high levels of triglycerides.

Cardiac catheterization: a diagnostic procedure in which specialized catheters are inserted into arteries and veins and advanced into the heart and its blood vessels.

Cardiovascular: relating to the heart and blood vessels.

Celecoxib (trade name, **Celebrex**): an anti-inflammatory drug used to treat arthritis.

Central nervous system (**CNS**): the brain and spinal cord.

Cerivastatin (trade name, **Baycol**): a statin that was taken off the market in 2001 because of a high risk of serious side effects.

Cholesterol: a waxy substance found in every cell of the body, which is important in the synthesis of various hormones, bile acids, and vitamin D. Circulates in the blood bound to special proteins called lipoproteins. High levels of certain lipoproteins (and low levels of high-density lipoproteins) are risk factors for developing atherosclerosis.

Cholestyramine (trade name, **Questran**): a medicine that belongs to a class called bile acid sequestrants. It is used to treat high levels of cholesterol.

Clot (also called a **thrombus**): blood that has solidified in a complex process involving formed blood elements called platelets and special proteins.

Coenzyme Q10 (**CoQ10**; also called **ubiquinone**): a molecule that is involved in energy generation by our cells. Levels are decreased by statins, and this may contribute to some statin side effects.

Cognitive function: our ability to think, remember, concentrate, and reason.

Congenital: something with which you are born.

Congestive heart failure: a condition in which the heart is unable to pump enough blood to meet the body's needs.

Coronary angiogram (also called **coronary angiography** or **coronary arteriography**): a diagnostic imaging procedure in which catheters are placed in the arteries supplying the heart, and dye is injected to determine whether or not there are blockages. The physician performing the coronary angiogram views and analyzes moving-picture X-ray images of the dye in the arteries.

Coronary artery: an artery supplying the heart muscle. Most people have two, called the right coronary artery and the left coronary artery. They are the first branches of the aorta after it arises from the left side of the heart.

Coronary artery bypass grafting (**CABG**; also called **coronary artery bypass surgery**): an operation in which the surgeon uses either leg veins or arteries from the arms and/or chest to bypass blocked arteries in the heart.

Coronary artery disease (**CAD**): disease of the

arteries that supply the heart muscle, caused most commonly by the buildup of atherosclerotic plaque.

Coronary heart disease (CHD): another term for coronary artery disease.

C-reactive protein (CRP; or hsCRP, for high-sensitivity CRP): a protein in the blood that is an indication of inflammation. An elevated CRP level is a risk factor for developing atherosclerosis.

Diabetes: a disease in which there is either insensitivity to or a lack of the hormone insulin. It is diagnosed by a blood test that reveals abnormally high levels of blood sugar. Diabetes is a major risk factor for developing atherosclerosis.

Diastole: that portion of the heart cycle when the heart is relaxed.

Diastolic blood pressure: the lower of the two blood pressure readings. It is the pressure in the arteries when the heart is relaxed.

Dyslipidemia (also called **dyslipoproteinemia**): abnormal levels of fats in the blood.

Echocardiogram (also called an **echocardiograph**): a test that uses sound waves to construct an image of the heart walls and valves in real time.

Electrocardiogram (also called **EKG** or **ECG**): a graphic display of the electrical activity of the heart; useful in diagnosing many heart conditions.

Embolus (plural, **emboli**; also called an **embolism**): a clot that has broken off from where it formed and traveled to another part of the body.

Enzyme: a specialized protein that speeds up chemical reactions.

Estrogen: one of the female reproductive hormones.

Estrogen replacement therapy (ERT): estrogen treatment of women after menopause.

Familial hypercholesterolemia: a rare, inherited disorder in which cholesterol is very elevated and in which there is a markedly increased risk for developing premature atherosclerosis. People with one dose of the gene that causes this disease have LDL cholesterols in the range of 300 to 400.

Fatty acids: Substances found in food that are building blocks of fats and are used by the body to generate energy.

Fatty streak: an early sign of atherosclerosis.

Fenofibrate (trade names, **Tricor, Trilipix**): a medicine used to treat high levels of triglycerides.

Fibric acid derivative (also called a **fibrate**): a class of medicines used to treat high triglycerides. When used in conjunction with a statin, may increase the risk of serious side effects.

Fibrous cap: a covering of scar tissue that walls off an atherosclerotic plaque and its contents from the bloodstream.

Fluvastatin (trade name, **Lescol**): a statin medicine used to treat high levels of LDL cholesterol.

Foam cells: white blood cells called **macrophages** that have gobbled up lots of lipid; found in atherosclerotic plaques.

Food and Drug Administration (FDA): a part of the US Department of Health and Human Services, it is responsible, among other things, for approving new prescription medications before they can be marketed in the United States.

Framingham Heart Study: a hallmark study begun in the late 1940s in which two-thirds of the adult population of Framingham, Massachusetts, participated. The ongoing study sought to determine the risk factors for atherosclerosis.

Gemfibrozil (trade name, **Lopid**): a medicine of the fibrate class used to treat high levels of triglycerides.

Glucose: a simple sugar that is used by the body to generate energy.

Hemorrhage: abnormal bleeding.

High-density lipoprotein (HDL): so-called good cholesterol; it can remove cholesterol from plaque. Higher levels are associated with a lower risk of atherosclerosis.

Hormone replacement therapy (HRT): estrogen and progesterone treatment of women after menopause.

Hypercholesterolemia: high blood levels of cholesterol.

Hyperglycemia: high levels of blood sugar (glucose).

Hyperlipidemia (also called **hyperlipoproteinemia**): elevation in the levels of blood fats; refers mainly to high concentrations of cholesterol and triglycerides.

Hypertension: high blood pressure. A risk factor for developing atherosclerosis.

Idiopathic: a fancy way of saying "We don't know what causes this."

Inferior vena cava: a large vein that returns blood from the lower body to the right side of the heart.

Insulin: a hormone made by the pancreas that regulates the level of glucose in the blood. High levels of insulin increase the risk of atherosclerosis.

Intima: the innermost layer of an artery. When the intima is damaged, cholesterol enters the blood vessel wall and starts to form a plaque.

Ischemia: a condition in which the blood supply to an organ, such as the heart, is insufficient for its needs at that point in time.

Ischemic heart disease (IHD): a disease caused by the buildup of atherosclerotic plaque in the arteries supplying the heart, depriving the organ of oxygen-laden blood.

JUPITER trial: a study that compared rosuvastatin (Crestor) to placebo in people with normal levels of LDL cholesterol but increased hsCRP.

Left anterior descending artery: one of the two major branches of the left coronary artery.

Left atrium: the upper, or receiving, chamber on the left side of the heart. It collects oxygenated blood coming from the lungs and directs it into the left ventricle.

Left circumflex artery: one of the two major branches of the left coronary artery.

Left ventricle: the chamber on the left side of the heart that pumps oxygenated blood into the aorta, from whence it is distributed to all the cells of the body.

Lipid: another word for blood fat.

Lipoprotein: a molecule made when lipids join to

a specialized protein, making that fat soluble in the blood.

Low-density lipoprotein (LDL): so-called bad cholesterol. High levels are a risk factor for developing atherosclerosis (more so in men than in women).

Lumen: the opening in an artery or vein through which blood flows.

Macrophage: a specialized white blood cell that can ingest bacteria or other harmful substances like oxidized LDL cholesterol.

Magnetic resonance imaging (MRI): a diagnostic test that uses magnetic energy to visualize the inside of the body.

McArdle's disease: a rare metabolic disease characterized by muscle pain and weakness after exercise. It may be unmasked by taking statins.

Mediterranean diet: the diet that was traditionally consumed by people living around the Mediterranean Sea. It is rich in fruits, vegetables, olive oil, legumes (beans), whole grains, and seafood, and low in meat.

Menopause: the cessation of menstruation for one year, after which a woman is said to be postmenopausal. In the United States, the average age at which this occurs is fifty-two.

Menses (menstruation): the monthly shedding of blood by the uterus during a woman's reproductive years.

Metabolic syndrome: a clustering of risk factors that greatly increases the risk of developing atherosclerosis. It is diagnosed if three out of the following five conditions are present: abdominal obesity, high blood pressure, high triglycerides, low HDL cholesterol, and elevated fasting blood glucose.

Mitochondria: microscopic energy factories found in all of our cells.

Mitochondrial myopathy: a condition that may be inherited or acquired in which muscle damage is caused by malfunction of the mitochondria.

Mitral valve: a one-way heart valve located between the left atrium and the left ventricle.

Myalgia: muscle pain.

Myasthenia gravis: a disease that features variable muscle weakness and fatigability.

Myelin sheath: a layer of insulation around nerves that is vital for their proper functioning. Certain diseases such as multiple sclerosis are associated with damage to the myelin sheath.

Myocardial infarction (heart attack): death of heart muscle due to interruption of its blood supply; caused most often by rupture of a plaque with clot formation that totally blocks blood flow through the affected coronary artery.

Myocardial ischemia: a condition in which the blood supply to the heart is not sufficient for its needs.

Myoglobin: a protein found in muscle. It is released into the bloodstream when muscle is damaged.

Myopathy: any muscle abnormality.

Myotonic dystrophy: adult-onset muscular dystrophy. It is characterized by muscle wasting and weakness. People with this disease may also have cataracts and defects in the heart's electrical system.

Neuropathy: damage to nerves.

Niacin: a B vitamin that in high doses raises HDL cholesterol, lowers triglycerides, and lowers LDL cholesterol; marketed as a prescription medication under the name **Niaspan**.

Nitrates: a class of medicines used to treat angina. Nitrates dilate blood vessels and decrease the work of the heart, thereby improving supply-demand imbalance.

Nitroglycerin: the most commonly prescribed medicine to treat angina.

Obesity: a body mass index of 30 or more.

Omega-3 fatty acids: polyunsaturated fats found in fish, walnuts, flaxseed oil, and canola oil that have anti-inflammatory properties. Those found in fish seem to protect against sudden cardiac death. In high doses, the fish-derived omega-3s lower triglyceride levels.

Omega-6 fatty acids: polyunsaturated fats found in safflower, corn, and soybean oils, among others. High intake of omega-6 fatty acids is thought to promote inflammation and therefore might increase the risk of atherosclerosis.

Osteoporosis: a condition in which bones thin and become more prone to fracture. It affects women more than men, particularly after menopause.

Oxygen: an element that is necessary for life. It is carried by the red blood cells in our arteries.

Paresthesia: an abnormal sensation such as numbness, tingling, or pins and needles.

Percutaneous coronary intervention (PCI): a procedure in which specialized catheters and devices called stents are placed in a narrowed coronary artery to increase the size of the lumen, thereby improving blood supply to the heart muscle. The same type of procedure can be used in other arteries; for example, those leading to the brain and to the legs.

Peripheral nervous system (**PNS**): all the nerves outside the central nervous system. The PNS is divided into the autonomic nervous system and the somatic nervous system.

Placebo: a sham or fake treatment used in the most scientifically valid studies to see if a medicine or procedure is effective.

Plaque: the name given to a complex material composed of foam cells, smooth muscle cells, cholesterol, scar tissue, and a fibrous cap that builds up in arteries affected by atherosclerosis.

Platelet: a cell fragment which plays a key role in blood clotting.

Polyneuropathy: damage to multiple nerves.

Pravastatin (trade name, **Pravachol**): a statin medicine used to treat high levels of LDL cholesterol.

Professional medical associations (**PMAs**): groups such as the American Medical Association, the American Heart Association, the American College of Cardiology, and so forth, which are influential in promulgating guidelines for physicians to follow and in providing professional educational conferences among other activities.

Progesterone: one of the female reproductive hormones.

Protein: one of the major food groups and a type of

molecule that is found throughout the body. Proteins contain compounds called amino acids, which are made up of carbon, hydrogen, oxygen, and nitrogen.

Pulmonary: relating to the lungs.

Pulmonary artery: the artery that leaves the right side of the heart and brings venous blood to the lungs for reoxygenation.

Pulmonary vein: a blood vessel in the lung that carries oxygenated blood to the left atrium.

Pulmonic valve: a one-way heart valve between the right ventricle and the pulmonary artery.

Randomized, Placebo-Controlled, Double-Blind Trial: in this type of trial, an active drug is compared to an indistinguishable placebo in groups that have similar levels of risk. Neither the people taking the drug/placebo, nor the investigators, know who is getting what until the study is ended.

Red rice yeast: a traditional Chinese herbal supplement that can lower LDL cholesterol because it contains lovastatin.

Rhabdomyolysis: severe breakdown of muscle tissue. A rare side effect of statins, rhabdomyolysis may lead to kidney failure and death. Usually causes severe muscle pain and weakness.

Right atrium: the upper chamber on the right side of the heart. It collects venous blood from around the body.

Right ventricle: the pumping chamber on the right side of the heart. It pumps venous blood to the lungs, where the blood takes up oxygen.

Risk factor: any characteristic that increases one's

risk of developing a disease, such as smoking or high blood pressure in the case of atherosclerosis.

Rosuvastatin (trade name, **Crestor**): the statin used in the JUPITER study.

Seven Countries Study: a landmark study begun in the 1950s by Dr. Ancel Keys that correlated dietary patterns with the risk of heart disease and other health problems.

Simvastatin (trade name, **Zocor**): a statin medicine used to treat high levels of LDL cholesterol.

Somatic nervous system: the division of the peripheral nervous system that controls voluntary muscle movements.

Statins: medicines that are effective in lowering high levels of LDL cholesterol and in lowering the risk of atherosclerosis in certain populations.

Stenosis: a narrowing or obstruction in a blood vessel or heart valve.

Stent: a tube, usually made up of metal or polymers, which is inserted into a narrowed artery, after a balloon has been used to expand the obstructed area (angioplasty).

Stroke: death of brain cells due to interruption of the blood supply by a clot in an artery. Another cause of stroke is a sudden hemorrhage into the brain.

Sudden cardiac death: death that occurs within minutes when the heart stops beating or beats too rapidly and inefficiently to allow blood to circulate.

Systole: the part of the cardiac cycle when the heart is contracting.

Testosterone: a male reproductive hormone; also found in women but in lesser amounts.

Thrombosis: clot formation when this should not be occurring.

Thrombus (plural, **thrombi**): a clot.

Tricuspid valve: a one-way heart valve between the right atrium and the right ventricle.

Triglyceride: a blood fat found mainly in VLDL cholesterol, which, when elevated, is a risk factor for developing atherosclerosis, particularly in women.

Valve: there are four of these in the human heart. They keep the blood flowing in the proper direction.

Vein: a blood vessel that carries blood that has given up oxygen and taken up carbon dioxide from cells in the body.

Ventricle: the heart's pumping chamber. In mammals, there are two ventricles, the right and the left.

Very-low-density lipoprotein (VLDL): the main carrier of triglycerides.

Vitamin D: a vitamin that is important in maintaining bone health and regulating the level of calcium in the blood. It can be produced by skin cells after exposure to sunlight.

Testosterone: a male reproductive hormone; also found in women but in lesser amounts.

Thrombosis: clot formation (when this should not be occurring)

Thrombus: a clot; thrombi: clots

Tricuspid valve: a one-way heart valve between the right atrium and the right ventricle.

Triglyceride: a type of fat. A high level of VLDL cholesterol, when elevated, is a risk factor for developing atherosclerosis, particularly in women.

Valve: there are four of these in the human heart. They keep the blood flowing in the proper direction.

Vein: a blood vessel that carries blood that is low in oxygen and picks up carbon dioxide from cells in the body.

Ventricle: the heart's pumping chambers; it pumps... their walls work to... the right and the left.

Very-low-density lipoprotein (VLDL): the main carrier of triglycerides.

Vitamin D: a vitamin that is important in maintaining and health and regulating the level of calcium in the blood. It can be produced by skin with exposure to sunlight.

ENDNOTES

Chapter 2: When Statins Help Most, and When They May Not Help at All

1. R. Angelmar, "The Rise and Fall of Baycol/Lipobay," *Journal of Medical Marketing* 7, no. 1 (January 2007): 77–88.

2. K. K. Ray, et al., "Statins and All-Cause Mortality in High Risk Primary Prevention: A Meta-Analysis of 11 Randomized Control Trials Involving 65,229 Participants," *Archives of Internal Medicine* 170, no. 12 (June 28, 2010): 1024–31.

Chapter 3: Common Side Effects of Statins: Cautionary Tales

1. L. Marcoff and P. Thompson, "The Role of Coenzyme Q10 in Statin-Associated Myopathy," *Journal of the American College of Cardiology* 49, no. 23 (June 12, 2007): 2231–37.

2. S. Franc, et al., "A Comprehensive Description of Muscle Symptoms Associated with Lipid-Lowering Drugs," *Cardiovascular Drugs and Therapy* 17, nos. 5–6 (September–November 2003): 459–65.

3. P. S. Phillips, et al., "Statin-Associated Myopathy with Normal Creatine Kinase Levels," *Annals of Internal Medicine* 137, no. 7 (October 1, 2002): 581–85.

4. D. Graham, et al., "Incidence of Hospitalized Rhabdomyolysis in Patients Treated with Lipid Lowering Drugs," *Journal of the American Medical Association* 292 (December 1, 2004): 2585–90.

5. S. Jamil and P. Iqbal, "Rhabdomyolysis Induced by a Single Dose of a Statin," *Heart* 90, no. 1 (January 2004): e3 doi:10.1136/heart.90.1.e2.

6. A. Sorokin, et al., "Rhabdomyolysis Associated with Pomegranate Juice Consumption," *American Journal of Cardiology* 98, no. 5 (September 1, 2006): 705–6.

7. L. Lilja, K. T. Kivistö, and P. J. Neuvonen, "Grapefruit Juice–Simvastatin Interaction: Effect on Serum Concentrations of Simvastatin, Simvastatin Acid, and HMG-CoA Reductase Inhibitors," *Clinical Pharmacology and Therapeutics* 64, no. 5 (November 1998): 477–83.

8. Medicines Adverse Reactions Committee of the New Zealand Medicines and Medical Services Safety Authority, *Adverse Reaction Reporting and IMMP: Minutes of the 114th Medicines Adverse Reactions Committee Meeting, Statins and Tendonopathy,* June 26, 2003. Available from URL www.medsafe.govt.nz/profs/adverse/Minutes114.htm, accessed August 23, 2010.

9. I. Marie, et al., "Tendinous Disorders Attributed to Statins: A Study on Ninety-six Spontaneous Reports in the Period 1990–2005 and Review of the Literature,"

Arthritis & Rheumatism 59, no. 3 (March 15, 2008): 367–72.

10. A. Beri, F. C. Dwamena, and B. A. Dwamena, "Association Between Statin Therapy and Tendon Rupture: A Case-Control Study," *Journal of Cardiovascular Pharmacology* 53, no. 5 (May 2009): 401–4.

11. K. Harada, S. Tsuruoka, and A. Fujimura, "Shoulder Stiffness: A Common Adverse Effect of Statins in Women?," *Internal Medicine* 40, no. 8 (August 2001): 817–18.

12. M. S. Beattie, et al., "Association of Statin Use and Development and Progression of Hip Osteoarthritis in Elderly Women," *Journal of Rheumatology* 32, no. 1 (January 2005): 106–110.

13. L. Perger, et al., "Fatal Liver Failure with Atorvastatin," *Journal of Hepatology* 39, no. 6 (December 2003): 1096–97.

14. A. Grieco, et al., "Acute Hepatitis Caused by a Natural Lipid-Lowering Product," *Journal of Hepatology* 50, no. 6 (June 2009): 1273–77.

15. M. Muldoon, et al., "Effects of Lovastatin on Cognitive Function and Psychological Well-Being," *American Journal of Medicine* 108, no. 7 (May 2000): 538–47.

16. M. Muldoon, et al., "Randomized Trial of the Effects of Simvastatin on Cognitive Functioning in Hypercholesterolemic Adults," *American Journal of Medicine* 117, no. 11 (December 1, 2004): 823–29.

17. D. Gaist, et al., "Statins and the Risk of Polyneuropathy," *Neurology* 58, no. 9 (May 14, 2002): 1333–37.

18. R. Edwards, K. Star, and A. Kiuru, "Statins, Neuromuscular Degenerative Disease and an Amyotrophic Lateral Sclerosis–like Syndrome: An Analysis of Individual Case Safety Reports from Vigibase," *Drug Safety* 30, no. 6 (2007): 515–25.

19. J. Shepherd, et al., "Pravastatin in Elderly Individuals at Risk of Vascular Disease (PROSPER): A Randomised Controlled Trial," *Lancet* 360, no. 9346 (November 23, 2002): 1623–30.

20. M. Bertagnolli, et al., "Statin Use and Colorectal Adenoma Risk: Results from the Adenoma Prevention with Celecoxib Trial," *Cancer Prevention Research* 3, no. 5 (May 2010): 588–96.

21. M. Sabatine, et al., "High-Dose Atorvastatin Associated with Worse Glycemic Control: A PROVE-IT TIMI-22 Substudy," *Circulation* 110, Supplement III (2004): 834.

22. P. Ridker, et al., "Rosuvastatin to Prevent Vascular Events in Men and Women with Elevated C-Reactive Protein," *New England Journal of Medicine* 359, no. 21 (November 20, 2008): 2195–2207.

23. N. Sattar, et al. "Statins and Risk of Incident Diabetes: A Collaborative Meta-Analysis of Randomised Statin Trials," *Lancet* 375, no. 9716 (February 27, 2010): 735–42.

24. J. Hippisley-Cox and C. Coupland, "Unintended Effects of Statins in Men and Women in England and Wales: Population Based Cohort Study Using the QResearch Data Base," *British Medical Journal* 340 (May 20, 2010): c2197.

25. M. B. Westover, et al., "Statin Use Following Intracerebral Hemorrhage: A Decision Analysis," *Archives of Neurology* 68, no. 5 (May 2011): 573–79.

26. R. J. Edison and M. Muenke, "Mechanistic and Epidemiologic Considerations in the Evaluation of Adverse Birth Outcomes Following Gestational Exposure to Statins," *American Journal of Medical Genetics* 131A, no. 3 (December 15, 2004): 287–98.

27. Pfizer Inc., "Pfizer's new chewable Lipitor for children receives European Commission approval," *News-Medical.net,* July 7, 2010, www.news-medical .net/news/20100707/Pfizers-new-chewable-Lipitor-for-children-receives-European-Commission-approval .aspx.

Chapter 4: Why Can't a Woman Be More Like a Man? Gender Differences and Statin Use

1. *The Inclusion of Women in Clinical Trials: Policies for Population Subgroups,* Report of the Institute of Medicine (1993).

2. J. Shepherd, et al., "Prevention of Coronary Heart Disease with Pravastatin in Men with Hypercholesterolemia: West of Scotland Coronary Prevention Study Group," *New England Journal of Medicine* 333, no. 20 (November 16, 1995): 1301–7.

3. J. Downs, et al., "Primary Prevention of Acute Coronary Events with Lovastatin in Men and Women with Average Cholesterol Levels: Results of AFCAPS/ TexCAPS," *Journal of the American Medical Association* 279, no. 20 (May 27, 1998): 1615–22.

4. P. Sever, et al., "Prevention of Coronary and Stroke Events with Atorvastatin in Hypertensive Patients Who Have Average or Lower-Than-Average Cholesterol Concentrations, in the Anglo-Scandinavian Cardiac Outcomes Trial—Lipid Lowering Arm (ASCOT-LLA): A Multicentre Randomised Controlled Trial," *Lancet* 361, no. 9364 (April 5, 2003): 1149–58.

5. Lozano, Mario, "Class Action Filed Against Pfizer Over Marketing of Lipitor," *Legal News Watch*, September 28, 2009, www.legalnewswatch.com/622/class-action-filed-against-pfizer-over-marketing-of-lipitor, (accessed December 2, 2011).

6. Light, Donald, "How Reducing Negligible Risks Drives Up Health Costs," December 12, 2008, www.scienceprogress.org/2008/12/how-reducing-negligible-risks-drives-up-health-costs (accessed December 2, 2011).

7. P. Ridker, et al., "Rosuvastatin to Prevent Vascular Events in Men and Women with Elevated C-Reactive Protein," *New England Journal of Medicine* 359, no. 21 (November 20, 2008): 2195–2207.

8. S. Mora, et al., "Statins for the Primary Prevention of Cardiovascular Events in Women with Elevated High-Sensitivity C-Reactive Protein or Dyslipidemia: Results from the Justification for the Use of Statins in Prevention: An Intervention Trial Evaluating Rosuvastatin (JUPITER) and Meta-Analysis of Women from Primary Prevention Trials," *Circulation* 121, no. 9 (March 9, 2010): 1069–77.

9. M. de Lorgeril, et al., "Cholesterol Lowering, Cardiovascular Diseases, and the Rosuvastatin-JUPITER Controversy: A Critical Reappraisal," *Archives of Internal Medicine* 170, no. 12 (June 28, 2010): 1032–36.

10. P. Chan, et al., *New England Journal of Medicine* (Correspondence) March 5, 2009; 360: 1039.

11. Y. Cui, et al., "Non-High-Density Lipoprotein Cholesterol Level as a Predictor of Cardiovascular Disease Mortality," *Archives of Internal Medicine* 161, no. 11 (June 11, 2001): 1413–19.

Chapter 5: So What Am I to Do? Practical Lifestyle Approaches to Heart Health

1. A. Keys, et al., "The Seven Countries Study: 2,289 Deaths in 15 Years," *Preventive Medicine* 13, no. 2 (1984): 141–54.

2. A. Keys, et al., "The Diet and 15-Year Death Rate in the Seven Countries Study," *American Journal of Epidemiology* 124, no. 6 (December 1986): 903–15.

3. M. de Lorgeril, et al., "The 'Diet-Heart' Hypothesis in Secondary Prevention of Coronary Heart Disease," *European Heart Journal* 18, no. 1 (January 1997): 14–18.

4. M. de Lorgeril, et al., "Mediterranean Diet, Traditional Risk Factors, and the Rate of Complications After Myocardial Infarction: Final Report of the Lyon Diet Heart Study," *Circulation* 99, no. 6 (February 16, 1999): 779–85.

5. www.americanheart.org/presenter; html?identifier-4655, (accessed June 19, 2010).

6. P. Mitrou, et al., "Mediterranean Dietary Pattern and Prediction of All-Cause Mortality in a U.S. Population: Results from the NIH-AARP Diet and Health Study," *Archives of Internal Medicine* 167, no. 22 (December 10, 2007): 2461–68.

7. L. A. Ferrara, et al., "Olive Oil and Reduced Need for Antihypertensive Medications," *Archives of Internal Medicine* 160, no. 6 (March 27, 2000): 837–42.

8. D. Jenkins, et al., "Effects of a Dietary Portfolio of Cholesterol-Lowering Foods Vs. Lovastatin on Serum Lipids and C-Reactive Protein," *Journal of the American Medical Association* 290, no. 4 (July 23, 2003): 502–510.

9. R. Estruch, et al., "Effects of a Mediterranean-Style Diet on Cardiovascular Risk Factors: A Randomized Trial," *Annals of Internal Medicine* 145 (2006): 1–11.

10. M. Fitó, et al., "Effect of a Traditional Mediterranean Diet on Lipoprotein Oxidation," *Archives of Internal Medicine* 167, no. 11 (June 11, 2007): 1195–1203.

11. I. Shai, et al., "Weight Loss with a Low-Carbohydrate, Mediterranean, or Low-Fat Diet," *New England Journal of Medicine* 359, no. 3 (July 17, 2008): 229–41.

12. S. Weinberg, "The Diet-Heart Hypothesis: A Critique," *Journal of the American College of Cardiology* 43, no. 5 (2004): 731–33.

13. "Egg, whole, raw, fresh," *Self Nutrition Data*, http://nutritiondata.self.com/facts/dairy-and-egg-products/111/2 (accessed July 30, 2010).

14. D. J. McNamara, "Dietary Cholesterol and Atherosclerosis," *Biochimica et Biophysica Acta* 1529, nos. 1–3 (December 15, 2000): 310–20.

15. J. S. Foer, *Eating Animals* (New York: Little, Brown and Company, 2009), 47.

16. A. N. DeMaria, "Eat Food, Not Very Much, Mostly Plants," *Journal of the American College of Cardiology* 55, no. 20 (May 18, 2010): 2288–89.

17. M. Pollan, *In Defense of Food: An Eater's Manifesto* (New York: Penguin Press, 2008), 1.

Chapter 6: The Chinese Got There First: Red Rice Yeast and the Dawn of the Statin Era

1. L. Slutsker, et al., "Eosinophilia-Myalgia Syndrome Associated with Exposure to Tryptophan from a Single Manufacturer," *Journal of the American Medical Association* 264, no. 2 (July 11, 1990): 213–17.

2. S. P. Zhao, et al., "Xuezhikang, an Extract of Cholestin, Reduces Cardiovascular Events in Type 2 Diabetes Patients with Coronary Heart Disease: Subgroup Analysis of Patients with Type 2 Diabetes from China Coronary Secondary Prevention Study (CCSPS)," *Journal of Cardiovascular Pharmacology* 49, no. 2 (February 2007): 81–84.

3. U.S. Food and Drug Administration, "FDA Warns Consumers to Avoid Red Yeast Rice Products Promoted on Internet as Treatments for High Cholesterol Products found to contain unauthorized drug," U.S. Department of Health & Human Services, August 9, 2007, www.fda.gov/NewsEvents/Newsroom/

PressAnnouncements/2007/ucm108962.htm,
(accessed December 2, 2011).

4. R. Y. Gordon, et al., "Marked Variability of
Monacolin Levels in Commercial Red Rice Yeast
Products," *Archives of Internal Medicine* 170, no. 19
(October 25, 2010): 1722–27.

Chapter 7: Big Pharma, the FDA, and the Medical Profession: An Unholy, Very Lucrative Alliance

1. D. Katz, A. L. Caplan, and J. F. Merz, "All Gifts
Large and Small: Toward an Understanding of the
Ethics of Pharmaceutical Industry Gift-Giving,"
American Journal of Bioethics 3, no. 3 (Summer 2003):
39–46.

2. Association of American Medical Colleges,
"The Scientific Basis of Influence and Reciprocity: A
Symposium," https://services.aamc.org/Publications/
showfile.cfm?file=version106.pdf&prd_id-215&prv_
id-262&pdf_id=106 (accessed June 11, 2010).

3. J. E. Bekelman, Y. Li, and C. P. Gross, "Scope
and Impact of Financial Conflicts of Interest in
Biomedical Research," *Journal of the American
Medical Association* 289, no. 4 (January 22–29, 2003):
454–65.

4. M. Angell, "Big Pharma, Bad Medicine," *Boston Review,* May–June 2010, http://bostonreview.net/
BR35.3/angell.php.

5. Information Please Database, "The Tuskegee
Syphilis Experiment," *Infoplease,* 2007, http://www
.infoplease.com/ipa/A0762136.html (accessed June 22,
2010).

6. Fauber, John, "Doctors' role in drug studies criticized," *JSOnline*, May 30, 2010, www.jsonline.com/features/health/95198129.html (accessed June 14, 2010).

7. U. A. Liberman, et al., "Effect of Oral Alendronate on Bone Mineral Density and the Incidence of Fractures in Postmenopausal Osteoporosis: The Alendronate Phase III Osteoporosis Treatment Study Group," *New England Journal of Medicine* 333, no. 22 (November 30, 1995): 1437–43.

8. D. M. Black, et al., "Bisphosphonates and Fractures of the Subtrochanteric or Diaphyseal Femur," *New England Journal of Medicine* 362, no. 19 (May 13, 2010): 1761–71.

9. S. Elad, et al., "Bisphosphonate-Related Osteonecrosis of the Jaw: Clinical Correlations with Computerized Tomography Presentation," *Clinical Oral Investigations* 14, no. 1 (February 2010): 43–50.

10. N. Yarom, et al., "Osteonecrosis of the Jaw Induced by Orally Administered Bisphosphonates: Incidence, Clinical Features, Predisposing Factors, and Treatment Outcome," *Osteoporosis International* 18, no. 10 (October 2007): 1363–70.

11. U.S. Food and Drug Administration, "Zolendronic Acid (Marketed as Reclast): Renal Impairment and Acute Renal Failure," *FDA Drug Safety Newsletter*, 2009, http://www.fda.gov/Drugs/DrugSafety/Drug SafetyNewsletter/ucm167883.htm#ZolendronicAcid MarketedasReclast:RenalImpairmentandAcuteLiver Failure (accessed June 21, 2010).

12. A. L. Herbst, H. Ulfelder, and D. C. Poskanzer,

"Adenocarcinoma of the Vagina: Association of Maternal Stilbestrol Therapy with Tumor Appearance in Young Women," *New England Journal of Medicine* 284, no. 15 (April 15, 1971): 878–81.

13. A. Goodman, J. Schorge, and M. F. Greene, "The Long-Term Effects of In Utero Exposures: The DES Story," *New England Journal of Medicine* 364, no. 22 (June 2, 2011): 2083–84, April 20, 2011 (10.1056/NEJMp1104409).

14. A. S. Kesselbaum, D. M. Studdert, and M. M. Mello, "Whistle-Blowers' Experiences in Fraud Litigation Against Pharmaceutical Companies," *New England Journal of Medicine* 362, no. 19 (May 13, 2010): 1832–39.

15. D. J. Rothman, et al., "Professional Medical Associations and Their Relationships with Industry: A Proposal for Controlling Conflicts of Interest," *Journal of the American Medical Association* 301, no. 13 (April 1, 2009): 1367–72.

16. Better Business Bureau, "American Heart Association," *Charity Reports Index,* February 2011, http://www.bbb.org/charity-reviews/national/health/american-heart-association-in-dallas-tx-173 (accessed June 19, 2010).

17. Center or Science in the Public Interest, "Non-Profit Organizations Receiving Corporate Funding," *Integrity in Science,* www.cspinet.org/integrity/nonprofits/american_heart_association.html (accessed June 18, 2010).

18. ERI Economic Research Institute, "Nonprofit Organization Information: American Heart

Association," *ERI Non-Profit Executive Compensation,* http://www.eri-nonprofit-salaries.com/index .cfm?FuseAction=NPO.Form990&EIN=135613797& Year=2007&Cobrandid=0&sourceid= (accessed June 19, 2010).

19. R. Micha, S. K. Wallace, and D. Mozaffarian, "Red and Processed Meat Consumption and Risk of Incident of Coronary Heart Disease, Stroke, and Diabetes Mellitus: A Systematic Review and Meta-Analysis," *Circulation* 121, no 21 (June 1, 2010): 2271–83.

20. Childs, Dan, "Is Wii Worthy of American Heart Association Accolade?" *ABC News,* May 17, 2010, http://abcnews.go.com/Health/HeartHealth/ wii-worthy-american-heart-assn-endorsement/ story?id=10663377 (accessed July 30, 2010).

21. T. B. Mendelson, et al., "Conflicts of Interest in Cardiovascular Clinical Practice Guidelines," *Archives of Internal Medicine* 171, no. 6 (March 28, 2011): 577–84.

22. S. Nissen, "Can We Trust Cardiovascular Practice Guidelines," *Archives of Internal Medicine* 171, no. 6 (March 28, 2011): 584–85.

23. Council of Medical Specialty Societies, *Code for Interaction with Companies,* March, 2011, http:// www.cmss.org/uploadedFiles/Site/CMSS_Policies/ CMSS%20Code%20for%20Interactions%20with%20 Companies%204-19-10.pdf (accessed July 30, 2010).

24. S. Wood, "Too stringent, or not enough? Doctors debate new ethics code for interactions with industry," theheart.org http://www.theheart.org/ article/1072861/print.do (accessed June 11, 2010).

25. R. Moynihan, I. Heath, and D. Henry, "Selling Sickness: The Pharmaceutical Industry and Disease Mongering," *British Medical Journal* 324, no. 7342 (April 13, 2002): 886–91.

Chapter 8: The Heart and Its Discontents: What Happens in Sickness and Health

1. C. Napoli, et al., "Fatty Streak Formation Occurs in Human Fetal Aortas and Is Greatly Enhanced by Maternal Hypercholesterolemia," *Journal of Clinical Investigation* 100, no. 11 (December 1, 1997): 2680–90.

2. *Morbidity and Mortality Weekly Report,* MMWR 48, no. 3 (1999): 649–56.

3. Borio, Gene, "Tobacco Timeline: The Twentieth Century 1900–1949—The Rise of the Cigarette," *Tobacco.org,* www.tobacco.org/resources/history/Tobacco_History20–1.html (accessed December 2, 2011).

Chapter 9: Clinical Research and the "Science" Being Used to Support Statin Use

1. The Coronary Drug Project Research Group, "The Coronary Drug Project: Design, Methods, and Baseline Results," *Circulation* 47, no. 3, supplement 1 (1973): 11—150.

2. P. L. Canner, et al., "Fifteen-Year Mortality in Coronary Drug Project Patients: Long-Term Benefit with Niacin," *Journal of the American College of Cardiology* 8, no. 6 (December 1986): 1245–55.

3. H. Buchwald, et al., "Effect of Partial Ileal

Bypass Surgery on Mortality and Morbidity from Coronary Heart Disease in Patients with Hypercholesterolemia," *New England Journal of Medicine* 323, no. 14 (October 4, 1990): 946–55.

4. J. F. Brensike, et al., "Effects of Therapy with Cholestyramine on Progression of Coronary Arteriosclerosis: Results of the NHLBI Type II Coronary Intervention Study," *Circulation* 69, no. 2 (February 1984): 313–24.

5. K. K. Ray, et al., "Statins and All-Cause Mortality in High-Risk Primary Prevention: A Meta-Analysis of 11 Randomized Control Trials Involving 65,229 Participants," *Archives of Internal Medicine* 170, no. 12 (June 28, 2010): 1024–31.

6. "Randomised Trial of Cholesterol Lowering in 4,444 Patients with Coronary Heart Disease: Scandinavian Simvastatin Survival Study Group," *Lancet* 344, no. 8934 (November 19, 1994): 1383–89.

7. "Prevention of Cardiovascular Events and Death with Pravastatin in Patients with Coronary Heart Disease and a Broad Range of Initial Cholesterol Levels: The Long-Term Intervention with Pravastatin in Ischaemic Disease (LIPID) Study Group," *New England Journal of Medicine* 339, no. 19 (November 5, 1998): 1349–57.

8. "MRC/BHF Heart Protection Study of Cholesterol Lowering with Simvastatin in 20,536 High-Risk Individuals: A Randomised Placebo-Controlled Trial," *Lancet* 360, no. 9326 (July 6, 2002): 7–22.

ACKNOWLEDGMENTS

I am deeply grateful to the following people for their advice and assistance: Naomi Rosenblatt; Barbara Lowenstein; Nancy Burke; my outstanding editor, Micki Nuding; Dr. Bernard Lown; Dr. Paul Thompson; the staff of the Women's Cardiac Center at the Miriam Hospital: Patty Shea Leary, RNP; Melissa Monteiro, and Maureen Dorego; my husband, Joe Avarista; and, as always, my patients, who are my first and best teachers.

INDEX